Design and Analysis of Clinical Nursing Research Studies

Colin R. Martin and
David R. Thompson

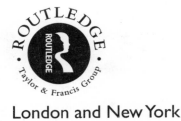

London and New York

First published 2000
by Routledge
11 New Fetter Lane, London EC4P 4EE

Simultaneously published in the USA and Canada
by Routledge
29 West 35th Street, New York, NY 10001

Routledge is an imprint of the Taylor & Francis Group

© 2000 Colin R. Martin & David R. Thompson

Typeset in Times and Gill Sans by
Prepress Projects Ltd, Perth, Scotland
Printed and bound in Great Britain by
Clays Ltd, St Ives plc

British Library Cataloguing in Publication Data
A catalogue record for this book is available
from the British Library

Library of Congress Cataloging in Publication Data
Martin Colin R., 1964–
    Design and analysis of clinical nursing research studies / Colin
R. Martin & David R. Thompson.
    p.   cm. – (Routledge essentials for nurses)
    Includes bibliographical references and index.
    ISBN 0-415-22598-1 (hb) – ISBN 0-415-22599-X (pb)
    1. Nursing – Research – Methodology. 2. Nursing – Research –
    Statistical methods. 3. Clinical medicine – Research –
    Methodology.
    I. Thompson, David R. II. Title. III. Series.
    [DNLM: 1. Clinical Nursing Research – methods. 2. Research
    Design – Nurses' Instruction. 3. Statistics – Nurses' Instruction.
    WY 20.5 m379bd 2000]
    RT81.5 .M27 2000
    610.73'07'2–dc21   00-034485

This book is dedicated to Caragh Brien-Martin,
Eloise Lily Robbins and Luke and Jack Thompson

Contents

Illustrations

Figures

Tables

Acknowledgements

We would like to thank the following friends and colleagues for their support and understanding in the writing of this volume and for their contribution to our ongoing research programmes: Dr Adrian Bonner, Pamela Canbaz, Sarah Ford, Mairwen Gale, Caroline Hollins, Corinna Petre and Rose Webster.

Foreword

The development of an evidence-based NHS is essential to improve and sustain high-quality clinical care and the appropriate organisation of health services. Nurses are vital to this effort, and nursing research must play its part in developing that evidence base.

Although there is a long research tradition in nursing, competing career options, lack of opportunity to develop research skills and the complex nature of institutional relationships between the service and higher education have constrained the development of nursing capacity and capability, particularly in clinical research. *Making a Difference*, the new national strategy for nurses, health visitors and midwives, signals a commitment to 'develop a strategy to influence the research and development agenda, to strengthen research capacity to undertake nursing, midwifery and health visiting research, and to use research to support nursing, midwifery and health visiting practice'.

There is clearly a need to develop expertise in clinical research, which will underpin the evidence base of the discipline and enhance the nursing contribution to both nursing and multidisciplinary research.

This text provides a step-by-step approach to the design of good-quality clinical nursing research and, using relevant examples, considers how this should be applied at both the design and analysis stages of all good studies. It demystifies the choice and application of statistical tests that give appropriate answers to important questions.

Poor research design and inappropriate methodology are far from uncommon in health-related research undertaken by *any* discipline. I certainly recommend this text to the nursing community, but also believe that it has relevance to many others about to embark on clinical research. Finally, David Thompson and Colin Martin are to be congratulated for producing a thoroughly readable and informative text.

Professor Sir John Pattison
Director of Research & Development
Department of Health

Chapter 1

Clinical research in nursing

Introduction

Developments in nursing as a research-based profession have continued apace over recent years. A key issue in terms of developing an evidence base in any discipline is the nature of the dominant philosophy underpinning the particular profession. The philosophy underlying the discipline must inevitably inform the direction and style of knowledge seeking undertaken *and* the accompanying methodology to execute this pursuit of evidence. In many areas of research, this does not present any real practical difficulties. In physics research, for example, a fundamental tenet underlying the accumulation of evidence is to adopt a scientific approach to the research enterprise, the methodology for which is clearly circumscribed within established design parameters. Nursing, on the other hand, presents us with a special case. The philosophy underlying nursing in terms of developing a research identity is not at all clear. This is due, in part, to the lack of clarity about what nursing represents regarding a dominant ideology; put simply, there is no clear consensus as to whether nursing is an 'art' or a 'science' (Thompson, 1998). Inevitably, this has led to the adoption of a wide variety of research methodologies applied to nursing research, all of which are legitimised by the presence of an ambiguous nursing ideology. Methodologies used in nursing research can be grouped into two distinctive camps, these being *qualitative* and *quantitative*.

Qualitative and quantitative approaches to nursing research

The distinction between qualitative and quantitative research in nursing is representative of a complex issue which will be simplified for the purposes of clarity and brevity. Broadly speaking, qualitative research takes the view that attempting to quantify the salient aspects of human experience in relation to health and disease represents a reductionist approach that cannot encapsulate the real matter of experience. As an example, a qualitative approach to understanding the process of recovery from surgery would focus on the context within which the individuals find themselves, the personal qualities of significant contacts during the period of treatment and the individuals' prior life experiences. It can be seen that these concepts would be difficult to measure numerically and to enter into a data analysis. This leads us then to a fundamental limitation of qualitative research in nursing, a lack of generality, replication and knowledge generation in terms of new theory.

Quantitative methodology addresses the criticisms of qualitative methodology by conducting studies that provide data in numerical form that can be entered into data analysis. Quantitative studies attempt to investigate a research question or 'hypothesis' by focusing on discrete and measurable aspects of an area of clinical and theoretical interest. The research question is therefore quantified. So, using the earlier example, in a quantitative study of recovery after surgery, we would be interested in measurable factors such as length of time in hospital, amount of anaesthetic given, type of anaesthetic given and number of previous procedures incurred by the patient. Further, we would want to be able to generalise the findings; so, using quantitative methodology, we may wish to compare different groups of patients defined by a particular characteristic such as diagnostic criteria and to compare the groups to investigate the differential effects of a treatment intervention. As the methodology used would be well circumscribed, replication of the study would be relatively simple.

A quantitative focus

It could be argued that an emphasis on the more qualitative aspects of nursing research in an era of evidence-based practice has led to an under-representation of quantitative methodology in present research endeavours. It is therefore crucial that nurses involved in quantitative research have available a text that covers experimental design and statistics in a context-sensitive manner. The following chapters will describe the design and statistical analysis of clinical nursing research studies using data from actual studies that have been conducted in the field. The breadth of the studies described will cover both general and mental health nursing research paradigms including data from multidisciplinary studies with a strong nursing contribution in the design and execution of the study. Although most statistical analyses are these days carried out on computer packages, these packages being discussed in Chapter 13, the emphasis within this text will be on the rationale for the tests used and their working out with reference to standard statistical tables included in the appendices. It is hoped that this approach will give the reader a more in-depth understanding of the philosophy and cerebral mechanics underpinning the tests, as well as providing the researcher with statistical independence when computer-based statistical packages are not available. The *applied* nature of the statistical tests described in this volume has been emphasised to indicate the ready applicability of the testing techniques to other appropriate clinical domains. The scope of the study designs and the associated statistical techniques covered has been intended to allow both the novice nurse researcher and the more seasoned professional nurse investigator to approach the design, execution and analysis of a study with confidence and optimism.

A common research language

An extremely useful by-product of nurses becoming familiar and proficient in the design, execution and analysis of quantitatively biased research projects is that it facilitates more readily collaborative ventures with other health disciplines such as medicine, clinical psychology, physiotherapy, etc. The reason for this salience is twofold. First, health disciplines other than nursing, and in particular medicine, have traditionally focused on quantitative approaches to the analysis of clinical material, this being dichotomous to the qualitative research approach which has been a traditional strength of the nursing profession. There is then a methodological issue involved in the failure to communicate between the two most influential professions involved in evidence-based patient care. Second, and more importantly for the future development of nursing as a research-based profession, the launch of the National Health Service (NHS) research and development (R&D) strategy *Research for Health* (Department of Health, 1991) stimulated increased interest in health-related research.

The NHS R&D strategy

This created new demands on the research community within and beyond the NHS and new opportunities for NHS staff to become involved in R&D. The importance of a sound research basis for nursing has been re-emphasised in the new strategy for nursing *Making a Difference* (Department of Health, 1999).

The aim of the NHS R&D strategy is to improve the health of the nation by promoting a knowledge-based health service in which clinical, managerial and policy decisions are based on sound research evidence. Although nursing needs to generate and extend its own body of knowledge through research, it is important that nursing research is seen as part of the broader scientific research community. The NHS R&D initiative offers nurses an ideal opportunity to engage in truly collaborative multidisciplinary and multiagency research, to demonstrate to others their own unique skills and distinct approach to research and to learn about the methods and approaches of others (Thompson, 1999). Further, the cross-fertilisation of skills from complementary disciplines allows freedom to develop more sophisticated research studies to address complex clinical questions previously occluded to single-discipline scientific enquiry (Martin *et al.*, 1998).

The research question

The key to the design of a good quantitative nursing study is to ask the right research question. Although this intrinsically crucial aspect of the research process may seem intuitively simple, a review of published literature across *all* disciplines will demonstrate that even seasoned researchers have not consistently formulated an appropriate research question and, consequently, have produced a flawed and lacklustre piece of work. Key identifying clues are often the use of 'esoteric', and usually inappropriate statistical tests to attempt to save a poorly conceived and/or executed study and a discussion section that bears no line of continuity to the introduction. Time spent *thinking* and *discussing* the question that we wish to address will *lead* the researcher to the correct methodology to implement the study. Essentially then, *all* quantitative research must begin with an appraisal of two key questions: 'I wonder if...' and 'I wonder why...'. These fundamental questions represent the skeleton of research design, the flesh being the hypotheses (formal research questions) and the skin being the methodology. Hopefully, this analogy illustrates the relative importance of formulating the research question; attempting to clothe a body of work with abstract statistics will in no way present a boneless and meatless study in a positive light. Time invested in considering the research question will pay dividends in getting work published and disseminated to the wider academic and clinical community.

Quantitative measurement of qualitative issues

Although much debate has taken place on the divide between qualitative and quantitative research in nursing, as a discipline nursing has come to represent a gestalt of the two approaches. This is easy to see why: patient contact focuses on the interpersonal aspects of health and ill-health in the recovery process, surely a *qualitative* issue. However, to influence policy, facts are required, and in terms of health care delivery and evaluation these are invariably based on *numeric*, and therefore *quantitative*, values. Considering qualitative and quantitative approaches as primary colours on the 'research palette', it is crucial to access all the 'shades of colour' between these extremes. One approach, the focus of this volume, is the quantification of qualitative data. Consider, as an example, clinical depression. There are a number of methods of assessing a person's depression. We may have an *opinion* about someone being depressed or not depressed; alternatively, we could conclude that the person is a little depressed or very depressed. The opinion is a subjective qualitative judgement, which may or may not be true; certainly, there is no reliable means of telling for sure. A *diagnosis* of depression is much the same, essentially a professional opinion. The diagnosis, like the opinion, is a qualitative judgement, prone to error and demonstrative of a restricted range of possibilities, i.e. depressed/not depressed or a limited range of labels describing levels of depression. It is, however, possible to measure depression quantitatively using a self-report measure such as the Beck Depression Inventory (Beck *et al.*, 1963).

This quantitative measurement of the qualitative experience of depression is enormously useful: it provides a larger range of possible levels of depression than the opinion or diagnosis; it allows comparison with a normal (i.e. non-depressed) population; it allows changes over time in levels of depression within an individual to be assessed accurately, quickly and reliably; it can inform treatment decisions and act as a measure of treatment efficacy; and it can be related to other measures of psychopathology, such as anxiety, to gain a more complete picture of the aetiology of depression within the individual. Further, comparison of defined groups of individuals on scores obtained on such quantitative measures can provide insights into the *nature* of depression and allow research questions to be asked that provide more answers to the causes of depression. This applies not only to psychological data, such as those obtained by the Beck Depression Inventory (BDI), but also to biological, biochemical, sociological and all behavioural data. The overarching theme between such diverse areas of speciality is that the data can be reduced to a numeric value. The advantage of obtaining a numerical value is that a statistical analysis can readily be made to tell whether there are significant differences between discrete treatment groups. This approach seeks to provide the researcher with factual evidence with which to test a *hypothesis*.

Hypothesis testing

If we wanted to compare the efficacy of two different treatments of *any* condition, it is desirable that the choice of the two treatments is based on a review of the available literature. This review would then inform us that we could reasonably expect one treatment to be more effective than the other based on this *prior* evidence. This expectation, based on the prior evidence that has been reviewed from the literature search, forms the basis of the experimental design and methodology that we would propose to use. This expectation regarding an outcome is common to all scientific exploratory studies and is known as the *hypothesis*. The hypothesis provides the formal focus from which the structure of the experimental method is defined. From the hypothesis, it is clear that *predictions* can be made that two treatments will differ in efficacy. The context within which health service research is constrained usually means that one new treatment or intervention is 'tested' against the established treatment/intervention. Traditionally, the epitome of this approach is embedded within the methodology of the randomised controlled trial.

The randomised controlled trial

The randomised controlled trial (RCT) has been the cornerstone of medical research, clinical trials in particular, for many years and has more recently become popular in testing hypotheses relating to nursing care. The basic premise of the RCT is that patients in one cohort are randomly allocated to two groups. One group, known as the control group, will receive the standard treatment; the second group, known as the treatment group, will receive the novel treatment. The efficacy of the new treatment will then be evaluated by a comparative analysis with the standard established treatment.

There are extreme limitations to the RCT approach to clinical research in nursing. It is likely that most nurse-led investigations will not be focusing on the effect of a drug treatment but will be examining an aspect of clinical nursing care. We may be interested in differences in recovery rates between two types of patient. For example, we may feel that mixed-sex wards have a greater impact on female patients' perceived level of anxiety than on male patients' perceived level of anxiety. It would not be appropriate, or possible, to conduct an RCT in this instance because it is sex that is the issue of interest within this particular environment (a mixed-sex ward), and it is impossible, after all, to randomise sex! The experimental designs that are applicable to these type of studies can be much more sophisticated than those of the RCT, the pay-off to these more elaborate studies being that the results can lay the foundations to a more theoretically meaningful examination of the issues central to the hypothesis.

Summary

This chapter has introduced the merits of the quantitative approach to clinical nursing research. Issues such as using quantitative methodology to develop a common research language with other disciplines involved in patient care have been discussed, as has the issue of quantifying qualitative data. The notions of the research question and the research hypothesis have been introduced. Limitations of the traditional medical approach to clinical research, in the form of the RCT, have been raised.

Chapter 2

Designing a clinical study

Introduction

Having decided upon a hypothesis to be tested, the next crucial phase is the design of the clinical study. To test the hypothesis that two distinct patient groups or two alternative treatments will be different, two vital factors need to be considered. First, it is crucial to consider the groups/ treatments that are being compared, and, second, what is to be measured; essentially, the numbers which will be entered into the statistical analysis. Because the researcher is exercising experimental control over the content of the patient groups or the types of treatment being compared, it is logical to conclude that the researcher is *manipulating* this particular variable. The variable that is being manipulated, such as group type or treatment type, is known as the independent variable (IV).

Considering the example of the mixed-sex ward in Chapter 1, the two groups of patients that are being compared are *male* patients and *female* patients. The IV in this instance is therefore *sex type*. Using the same example, having defined the two groups, it is then necessary to measure the effect of this manipulation; in this case, a measure of anxiety. However anxiety is measured, for example by a self-report questionnaire or by a biochemical measure such as serum cortisol, the score of anxiety on the questionnaire or the absolute amount of cortisol that is measured is known as the *dependent variable* (DV). This is obviously quite logical as the DV is literally dependent on the IV. The measure of anxiety expressed by each group is then compared by the use of a statistical test to find out whether male and female patients are significantly different in the terms of this measure of anxiety. It could be concluded that manipulating the IV caused the difference (if any were observed) in anxiety between the two groups. This would of course be exactly the same in the case of the IV being treatment type and the DV being a measure of outcome. Once the researcher has decided on a hypothesis to be tested and the choice of

IV and DV, the methodology can be formulated within the context of the research design.

Confounding variables

Having decided on the choice of IV and DV, the researcher will need to conduct a study that has a *rigorous* methodology. This rigour relates to the need to show that whatever differences are seen in the DV are purely a result of the manipulation of the IV and are not the result of some other uncontrolled or *confounding* variable. Confounding variables are the death knell of many a promising research study. For the most part, avoiding experimental confound lies in a good experimental design. Using the mixed-sex ward again as an example, having manipulated sex type, it was found that female patients were more anxious than male patients on a self-report measure of anxiety; this finding is fine as long as all *other* variables are controlled, the only differences between the two groups being the patients' sex. However, having come to this conclusion, what happens if closer inspection of all the patients' characteristics reveals that the male patients are generally much older than the female patients? It could no longer be concluded that the difference in anxiety observed between male and female patients was due to sex because it could be due to the difference in patient age between the two groups. In this respect, age has acted as a confounding variable because it was not controlled for in the experimental manipulation. There are of course a huge number of variables which are not germane to the study that is being designed that could *potentially* become confounding variables. It is possible to control for these *irrelevant* variables by the process of randomisation and subject matching which will be discussed later in this chapter.

Experimental design

There are essentially three types of experimental design that will be encountered in the clinical setting. These three design types afford differing degrees of control over subject/patient variables before a manipulation of the IV. The design types describe the way in which the subject or patient will be allocated to a particular experimental group.

The within-subjects design

The within-subjects design, also known as the repeated measures design, affords the most control of subject variables because the same subjects are used in each group. In the instance of the within-subjects design, the patient would undergo all treatment options. Alternatively, repeated observations may be made of the patient over the course of a treatment programme. It can be seen that if all patients were to be offered two treatments consistently in the same order the first treatment may have an effect on the efficacy of the second treatment. This situation, a systematic influence of the first condition on the second, is known as an order effect and is a prime source of experimental confound. Fortunately, effects of this kind are easy to control by the use of counterbalancing techniques. Counterbalancing simply means controlling the order in which treatments are presented to the patient, in this case half of a cohort of patients receiving treatment A first and the remaining patients receiving treatment B first. The purpose of counterbalancing is thus to balance these order effects over the course of the entire study. It may seem obvious, and indeed it is true to say, that the within-subjects design is not the most popular choice in clinical studies in which treatments such as novel pharmacological therapies are being introduced because the patient will undergo two treatment protocols with doubtful therapeutic justification. However, the within-subjects design has great utility where multiple observations are required to evaluate the effectiveness of a treatment over a period of time. An example of this would be the comparison of self-report depression scores before and after treatment. The within-subjects design can be extended to include more than two levels of the IV.

The matched-subjects design

The matched-subjects design is not usually encountered in clinical studies but is included here for completeness. The matched-subjects design attempts to emulate the degree of control offered by the within-subjects design over subject variables by matching subject variables as closely as possible without using the same subjects in each group. Often, this is accomplished by using sets of twins as subjects and allocating each twin to an alternative group. Even in the case of twins, and precluding some purely genetic research, it is not possible to match the individual's life experiences. Therefore, accepting the closest match of subjects, this design cannot control for subject variables as well as the within-subjects design.

The between-subjects design

An alternative to the within-subjects and matched-subjects designs is the between-subjects design, also known as the independent groups design. Acknowledging that rigorous control of subject variables is extremely difficult to achieve, the independent groups design splits the patient group into two distinct groups, usually on a random basis. Although the between-subjects design offers little control over subject variables, it has the advantage that it can be used and adapted in almost any clinical study. Indeed, the process of randomly allocating patients to each group does afford a degree of control of subject variables because, all other things being equal, subject attributes should be represented more or less equally in both groups. In effect, the process of randomisation allows patient differences to be balanced out across groups. Randomisation is particularly effective in clinical studies in which large numbers of patients are recruited. The between-groups design is, in fact, the basis of the randomised controlled trial (RCT) that was discussed in Chapter 1. The between-groups design can be extended to include more than two levels of the IV.

In terms of controlling subject variables, the within-subjects design offers the most effective control, followed by the matched-subjects design, with the between-subjects design being the least effective. However, the between-subjects design offers the greatest degree of utility in the design and execution of clinical studies, and the randomisation procedure affords some protection from any potential confounding effect of subject variables.

The mixed-group design

The mixed-group design is a combination of the between-subjects and within-subjects designs. Essentially, there would be two IVs; one of these would be between subjects and the second would be within subjects. The mixed design is the least often encountered design in clinical studies, yet it provides a most useful and effective experimental platform to address more sophisticated types of research question. The following clinical example and rationale illustrate this. For many years there has been some evidence to support the notion that there is a genetic contribution to the aetiology of alcoholism. Much of this research has been based on the expression of physiological phenomena during the detoxification process. In essence, there is some evidence to suggest that alcoholics with a positive family history (FH⁺) of alcoholism experience more severe withdrawal symptomatology than alcoholics without a family history of alcoholism (FH⁻). The detoxification regime for alcohol dependency when conducted in an in-patient setting usually takes place over several days, usually between 5 and 7 days. Therefore, the expression of withdrawal symptomatology would be assessed over this period, thus entailing multiple observations of withdrawal phenomena. To test a hypothesis that FH^+ alcoholics would have more severe withdrawals from alcohol than FH^- alcoholics, withdrawal symptoms would necessarily have to be assessed over more than one observation point. For the purposes of clarity, let us suppose that we would assess withdrawals of all alcoholic patients on days 2 and 5 of detoxification, this representing a within-subjects observation. However, there are two groups of alcoholics being assessed (FH^+ and FH^-), a between-subjects observation. Therefore, to address this research question, a mixed design is necessary because the two groups of alcoholics will all be assessed for withdrawal symptomatology over a number of observations (in this case, two). Like the between-groups and the within-groups designs, the mixed-group design can be extended so that more than two levels of each IV can be used in the study.

Non-subject variables

Although the experimental designs highlighted above *explicitly* state the degree of control over subject variables and also inform the researcher on additional safeguards in the sphere of experimental control (i.e. randomisation), it is also important to control for non-subject-related variables to reduce the risk of an experimental confound. Non-subject-related variables refer to specific environmental influences that may influence the results of a study. These influences could be factors such as time of day or change of personnel. As an example, let us consider diabetes mellitus. Let us suppose that a new insulin is under trial which should, in theory, offer greater control of blood sugar levels than a standard insulin regime and that the patient cohort is *randomly* allocated to two groups, A (treatment) and B (control), in a *between-groups* design. If all group A patients had blood taken for blood sugar measurement at 11.00 a.m. and all group B patients had blood taken at noon, it would be impossible to say whether any significant difference in blood sugar control found was the effect of the novel treatment (group A) or was related to the difference in the time of day when the blood was taken as it is well established that blood sugar levels are influenced by circadian rhythms and thus naturally change during the course of the day. However, if half of group A and half of group B patients had blood taken at 11.00 a.m. and the remainder of groups A and B patients had blood taken at noon, then the influence of the circadian effect on blood sugar levels would be controlled for. This process is called *balancing* the design. Any difference that was then observed between groups A and B may then be more reliably concluded to be due to the effect of the novel insulin treatment. Alternatively, the process of *randomisation* that was illustrated earlier in this chapter to control for subject/patient variables can also be used as it is readily extended to non-subject variables. In this, patients from both groups would be randomly allocated to the two *blood-sampling times*, 11.00 a.m. and noon. Sufficiently larger numbers of subjects would be likely to result in a balanced design as probability factors would dictate that 'more or less' half of group A patients and half of group B patients would be allocated to the 11.00 a.m. blood-sampling time with the remainder (around 50 per cent) being randomly allocated to the noon blood-sampling time. Although a different methodology has been used, the result is a *balanced* design. This is not the end of the story, however, as a degree of common sense must also enter the methodological equation. Because the circadian effect on blood sugar is so well documented, and may well be an important factor in how the new insulin offers a treatment advantage, it would be a wise precaution, from a methodological rigour point of view, to have *all* the blood samples taken at 11.00 a.m. *or all* the blood samples taken at noon. This is because, although we may have previously controlled for *systematic* time of day effects, we can further claim, by standardising the time of blood sampling, that any difference between groups A and B is not under any influence of circadian effect. Essentially, the fewer non-subject variables that have to be controlled for, the better. In this example, the circadian effect need not be an issue simply by taking *all* the blood samples at the same time of day.

Scales of measurement

There are four different levels of DV measurement; the distinction being drawn because these levels of measurement partly inform the appropriate statistical test. These are:

- nominal;
- ordinal;
- interval;
- ratio.

The *nominal* scale is the weakest level of measurement. Numbers are used to classify behaviour/phenomena into different classes *without* implying that the classes are numerically related. Nominal scaling is a method of labelling qualitative phenomena with a numeric value.

Ordinal scaling is used when ranking data. In this case, the numbers do possess quantitative meaning. Consider a patient who is asked to rate the pain they may be experiencing on a 1–7 scale, where a score of 1 equates to minimal pain and a score of 7 equates to extreme pain. Obviously, a score of 6 would be considered to be more painful than a score of 2. However, because of the subjectivity of the rating, it would be impossible to say that the difference in pain between scores 2 and 3 is equivalent to the difference in pain between scores 6 and 7. The ordinal scale indicates the order of items of a particular attribute, but not their separations on the scale.

Interval scaling and *ratio* scaling can be considered to be the highest levels of scaling. Not only is the ordering of items on the scale known but also the relative separation of items on the scale. A classic example of interval scaling is temperature. It is clear that the temperatures 10°C, 20°C and 30°C represent increasing levels of heat, thus satisfying the criteria of an ordinal rating. However, it can also be concluded that the difference between 10°C and 20°C is the same as the difference between 20°C and 30°C (i.e. 10°C). The scale thus achieves an interval level of measurement. The main difference between an interval and ratio scale is that a ratio scale must have an absolute zero point. We can say that time measured in seconds has an absolute zero point and can thus be considered a ratio measurement. Temperature, on the other hand, could be measured in centigrade *or* Fahrenheit. Measured in centigrade, it is possible to have temperatures below a zero point (i.e. −5°C). Statistically, this difference between interval and ratio scales is not, for our purposes, too important because the data derived from these two scales are generally subjected to the same types of statistical test.

The key to understanding statistics is therefore inseparable from the study design. The type of statistics that are used to analyse the results of an investigation are always a function of the study design.

A brief summary thus far

To conduct a study, we may wish to compare two (or more) different forms of treatment or compare two (or more) different types of patient. In an experimental study, differentiating groupings in this way is often called experimental *manipulation*. The variable that we manipulate (i.e. treatment type or patient type) is called the *independent* variable. Obviously, this is merely half the story because, having manipulated the independent variable, we need to measure 'something' to be able to gain a set of data before performing any statistics. The 'something' that we measure is known as the *dependent* variable. The dependent variable could be an outcome measure of some sort or could be a psychological measure, such as depression, or a biochemical measure, such as serum serotonin level. The main point is that the dependent variable (DV) will invariably have (or be given) a numerical value and is contingent on the independent variable (IV). The DV can be measured on a limited number of scale types. The IV and the DV inform the type of statistical test that will be used in the analysis.

Chapter 3

The qualities and power of data

Introduction

In the previous chapter, the fundamental aspects of experimental design were explored; in particular, the meaning of experimental manipulation, *independent variables* (IV) and *dependent variables* (DV). Further, the distinction between scales of measurement were examined, these levels of measurement being *nominal*, *ordinal*, *interval* and *ratio*. The importance of these aspects of experimental design is, among other things, that they inform the choice of the particular statistical test that will be used to measure differences that may interest us (e.g. the effect of treatment).

However, it is also vital to be able to summarise data and characterise the value of a set of scores (the raw data and our DV). Why? Well, for one thing, it does not make sense to present the whole of a data set in a published piece of work because space is at a premium; second, not only does a summary figure describing a set of scores take up less space but it may also give clues to the shape of the distribution of a data set, which will be a consideration when choosing the type of statistical test to use. A useful metaphor is to think of experimental design in general and the raw data (DV scores/values) as the 'cake' and the statistical tests that will later be applied as the 'icing'. This metaphor serves to remind the investigator that no amount of fancy icing will cover up a badly prepared or ill-conceived cake. Essentially, it is crucial to understand the nature of our data and to be able to describe them adequately before applying a statistical test. Indeed, the statistical test itself is a very small, albeit crucial, aspect of the research enterprise. Putting this into context, it is possible broadly to describe two types of statistics. These are *descriptive* statistics and *inferential* statistics. Descriptive statistics are basically summaries and descriptions of the data without the application of any kind of statistical test. Descriptive statistics would therefore include measures of central tendency and dispersion or variation of scores around the mean and also the description of data in graphical form, such as in bar or pie charts (discussed in Chapter 11). Inferential statistics, as may be guessed from the name, allow some kind of inference to be made about causality in the data, usually following the argument that treatment A was better than treatment B or that patient group C recovered quicker than patient group D. This level of inference can only be achieved if the inference itself is made with some degree or level of certainty. Inferential statistics only enable statistical significance to be determined. They do not permit inferences to be made about causality. Causality may only be inferred from the experimental design. The statistical test is fundamentally grounded on the concept of degrees of certainty or probability and the statistical tests are correspondingly known as inferential statistics. The bulk of this chapter will focus on descriptive statistics because a knowledge of these lays the foundation for the inferential statistics that will be described in later chapters. Further, as will be seen in this chapter and those that follow, descriptive summary statistics are used in the calculation of inferential statistics and are a feature of *all* statistical tests.

Measures of central tendency

Certainly, one of the most important summary statistics that will be observed frequently in published clinical reports is the measure of central tendency. The most commonly used measures of central tendency are the *mean*, *median* and *mode*. Most people will remember these terms from school days, but we will recap as follows.

1   Mean. Often described as the 'average', the mean is found by adding together every score and then dividing this total by the number of scores. The mean is the most frequently reported measure of central tendency that will be observed in published studies.
2   Median. An alternative to the mean is the median. The median represents the mid-point score in the range of data from lowest to highest scores. In this respect, the median is even easier to find than the mean.
3   Mode. The mode is defined as the most frequently occurring score in the set of scores.

Choosing the measure of central tendency

The mean is the preferred measure of central tendency in a normally distributed *symmetrical* data set, i.e. most scores fall around the mean and evenly taper off from the mean with few very high and few very low scores. However, there may be circumstances when the data set is *asymmetrical* or *skewed*. A distribution of scores with a larger number of low scores than high scores around the mean is known as a *negatively skewed* distribution. Conversely, a distribution of scores with a larger number of high scores than low scores around the mean is known as a positively *skewed* distribution. This can happen when there are a number of extreme scores, essentially the presence of a small number of very high scores or, alternatively, very low scores. In the event of a skewed data set, the median may be a more useful measure of central tendency because it is not readily influenced by extreme scores. The mode has limited use as a measure of central tendency and is not frequently used in the presentation of research findings.

The data spread

Having decided on the summary statistic of choice of central tendency, usually but not exclusively the mean, the next important factor to consider is the *spread* of the data. The spread of the data refers to how the data fall away from the central measure, whether this be the mean or the median. The spread or *dispersion* of the data is indeed a vital descriptive statistic as it is used in conjunction with the mean to estimate whether there is a statistically significant difference between two conditions, as measured by the DV and circumscribed by the IV.

The data range

The primary estimate of the spread of the data set is the range of scores from lowest to highest. The *range statistic* is calculated by subtracting the lowest score in the data set from the highest. Although the range statistic is an extremely useful measure of data spread and also benefits from being extremely easy to calculate, it can be a potentially misleading statistic under certain circumstances. These circumstances primarily involve skewed data distributions or the presence of a few extremely high or low scores in an otherwise well-distributed data set. It is easy to see how these specific circumstances can lead to a misleading range score. Consider the following post-operative patient pain self-assessment scores which have been assessed on a 0 (no pain) to 100 (extreme pain) visual analogue scale (VAS):

45   52   54   57   63   64   67   69   71

The range statistic in this example is 26 (71 – 45). The range statistic in this example provides a useful index of data spread and summarises the data in terms of data dispersion very well. However, consider the same data as the example above but with the substitution of the lowest score by an extremely low score:

13   52   54   62   63   64   67   69   71

The range statistic in this example is 58 (71 – 13). The range statistic has been affected by the extremely low score and its usefulness as an index of data spread has been compromised merely by the presence of *just one* extremely low score. A method to minimise the influence of extreme scores on the range statistic is to calculate the range from the middle 50 per cent of scores only from lowest to highest. The lowest score is taken from the 25 per cent point of the range of scores, this point being called the *first quartile*. The highest score is taken from the 75 per cent point of the range of scores, this point known being as the *third quartile*. The first quartile score is then subtracted from the third quartile score to calculate the range statistic. As quartiles are used to define the range statistic in this instance, it is termed the *interquartile range*. Using the same data that were used to calculate the range statistic:

Quartile (%)	First (25%)					Third (75%)		
45	52	54	57	63	64	67	69	71

In this well-distributed example data set, the interquartile range is 13 (67 – 54).

Now consider the data set with the extremely low score:

Quartile (%)	First (25%)					Third (75%)		
13	52	54	62	63	64	67	69	71

In this example data set, which includes an extremely low score (13), the interquartile range is still 13 (67 – 54), as in the previous example. Contrasting the two range estimations, the range statistic and the interquartile range, it can be clearly seen that the interquartile range provides a degree of protection against the influence of extreme scores.

Although the range estimate and interquartile range are useful measures of spread, there are more sophisticated measures of spread which are used in statistical calculations. These will now be discussed.

Variance

Variance is the summary term used to describe the degree to which the value of each subject or patient score is distant from the mean. To provide an example, consider the data set in Table 3.1, which shows eight patients' systolic blood pressure observations.

The mean blood pressure score is obtained by adding all the blood pressure observations together and dividing by the total number of observations, thus:

$$\text{Mean score} = \frac{(160+100+120+110+130+140+150+130)}{8}$$

$$= \frac{1040}{8}$$

$$= 130$$

It is also appropriate at this stage to introduce mathematical notation for the purposes of brevity. The mathematical notation used in this volume is consistent with that of other statistical texts, therefore gaining a knowledge of mathematical notation at this stage will be an excellent precursor to future reading in this area.

An individual subject score is usually given the abbreviation X. The mean is abbreviated to $\overline{X}$. The total number of subjects or patients in a study, or in a particular treatment group, is given the symbol N. The sum of a set of values (i.e. total of subject/patient scores) is given the Greek letter sigma Σ, which means the sum of a set of numbers. Translating this to the above blood pressure mean score calculation, the mathematical notation would thus be:

$$\overline{X} = \frac{\Sigma X}{N}$$

Table 3.1 A dataset of patients' systolic blood pressure observations

Patient number	Systolic blood pressure (mmHg)
1	160
2	100
3	120
4	110
5	130
6	140
7	150
8	130

New notation will be introduced into the text from this point onwards, with a full explanation of the meaning of each new item as appropriate.

Continuing with the blood pressure estimations, deviation is calculated by subtracting the mean score from each patient's blood pressure measurement. Therefore:

Deviation $= X - \overline{X}$

The variances for each patient are tabulated as shown in Table 3.2.

A closer examination of the individual score variances reveals a problem if the deviation were summarised by simply adding the individual variances together; a total deviation score under this rubric would always result in zero because of the presence of negative deviation scores. The solution that is utilised to get around this difficulty is to square all of the deviations, then to sum them and *then* to divide this sum by the number of observations. This results in the *variance*, the mathematical notation being S^2, and is represented by:

$$S^2 = \frac{\sum \left(X - \overline{X}\right)^2}{N}$$

Again, using the blood pressure observations as an example, the variance is calculated (see Table 3.3).

Although the variance is calculated to be 350, this is not the whole story. It has been estimated that a more accurate variance figure can be calculated by dividing the total deviation score by the total number of observations *minus one observation*. This is a standard procedure for calculating the total variance and is utilised by most computer statistical packages. Thus:

Table 3.2 Patients' blood pressure variances I

Patient number	Systolic blood pressure (mmHg)	Mean	Deviation
1	160	130	30
2	100	130	−30
3	120	130	−10
4	110	130	−20
5	130	130	0
6	140	130	10
7	150	130	20
8	130	130	0

$$S^2 = \frac{\sum (X - \overline{X})^2}{N-1}$$

Therefore:

Total deviation = 2800

Variance   = 2800/7 = 400

In summary, the total deviation scores divided by the number of observations minus one gives the estimated variance, also known as the sample variance or estimated population variance. The total deviation score divided by the number of observations gives the population variance, also more simply referred to as the variance.

Standard deviation

The *standard deviation* is the most frequently presented measure of spread in results summary tables, usually accompanying the mean. The standard deviation is a function of the mean and, therefore, the variance. Indeed, the standard deviation is the square root of the variance and is expressed as S or, more usually, as SD. The standard deviation is expressed as thus:

$$S = \sqrt{\frac{\sum (X - \overline{X})^2}{N-1}}$$

Table 3.3 Patients' blood pressure variances II

Patient number	Systolic blood pressure (mmHg)	Deviation	Deviation squared
1	160	30	900
2	100	−30	900
3	120	−10	100
4	110	−20	400
5	130	00	000
6	140	10	100
7	150	20	400
8	130	00	000
Total			2800

Total deviation = 2800

Variance   = 2800/8 = 350

The normal distribution

Having outlined the measures of central tendency and spread, it is fairly clear that most case scores will fall close to the mean, with fewer scores being more extreme from the mean. The fundamental shape to this type of distribution of scores is a bell-like shape and, most importantly, it tends to reoccur in a broad variety of data sets, including psychological, physical and biological variables. It is known as the *normal distribution* and is shown in Figure 3.1.

A classic example of a normal distribution in relation to human variables is intelligence. Being symmetrical, the mean, median and mode will usually have similar values. The normal distribution is of fundamental importance to a number of the statistical tests described in later chapters. The normal distribution is also useful in describing data, particularly in relation to the standard deviation, because it is possible to quantify the proportion of scores that fall above and below a number of standard deviations on the normal distribution. It is possible to transform an individual case score that may be of interest to indicate the score's distance from the mean, which is measured in units of standard deviations. This transformation produces a *Z score* and is expressed as follows:

$$Z = \frac{X - \overline{X}}{S}$$

Probability

Inevitably, having conducted an investigation, a statistical test will be conducted on the DV scores to determine whether there is a *statistically*

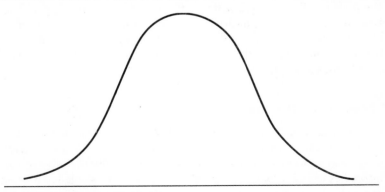

Figure 3.1 The normal distribution

significant difference between these scores as a function of the IV manipulation. Using the example of withdrawal symptomatology (DV) and family history status (IV) in alcohol-dependent individuals from Chapter 2, let us suggest the following summary data. On day 4 of withdrawal, the FH⁺ alcoholics have a mean withdrawal rating of 6.1 and the FH⁻ alcoholics have a mean withdrawal rating of 5.2. Although a descriptive examination of the data reveals that the FH⁺ alcoholics have a higher (more severe) mean withdrawal rating than FH⁻ alcoholics, how can we conclude that the difference between the groups is big enough for us to conclude that the difference is statistically significant? Irrespective of the fact that each design and data type utilises a different mathematical equation to compare differences, in all cases the determination of a *statistically significant* difference between groups is arbitrarily determined and is based on a probability estimate. This state of arbitrary inference is due to the reality of the situation that we may observe a large difference between groups yet this may still be down to a chance effect or rather *not* down to the IV manipulation. Therefore, statistical tests are determined to be statistically significant if it is highly likely that differences between DV scores are due to the experimental manipulation rather than chance factors. The arbitrary probability that has been established in the literature for a statistically significant difference between two or more sample means is 0.05. This figure, known as alpha or α, is based on the probability that out of twenty observations observed between sample means one of these observations will have been statistically significant by chance and is *not* due to the effect of the IV manipulation. The figure of 0.05 is therefore the function of 1 divided by 20. Because this is a probability estimation, 0.05 is prefixed with a *P* (probability). A figure of *P* at or *less than* 0.05 is deemed to be statistically significant. A *P*-value greater than 0.05 is deemed to indicate that there is no statistically significant difference between sample means. A *P*-value of 0.01 is often described as an indication of a *highly significant* difference between sample means; this would, of course, occur *by chance* in just 1 in 100 cases at this level.

Hypothesis testing

In most instances, of course, the researcher is testing a research question or 'hypothesis' based on a prediction. Therefore, in the alcohol-dependency example, the researcher might rationally predict that FH⁺ alcoholics will have more severe withdrawals than FH⁻ alcoholics because of genetic factors influencing the severity of withdrawal symptomatology.

The researchers' prediction that genetic factors will influence the severity of withdrawals between the two groups is known as an *alternate* or *experimental hypothesis*. There is, however, the possibility that any difference in severity between the two groups is purely down to chance variation in the withdrawal scores and is *not* due to any genetic effect associated with alcohol dependency; this is known as the *null hypothesis*.

Both types of hypothesis are important because, on the basis of the statistical test, we can reject the *null hypothesis* if $P = 0.05$ or $P < 0.05$ and therefore accept the *alternate* or *experimental hypothesis*. However, if $P > 0.05$, then the *alternate* or *experimental hypothesis* is rejected and the *null hypothesis* is accepted.

Type I and type II errors

Accepting that determining a statistically significant difference between groups is based on the probability that there is a real difference between groups as a function of the IV manipulation, there will be rare instances when the null hypothesis is rejected when it is actually correct. This is known as a *type I* error. As such, the probability of commiting a type I error is determined by the P-value determined. Therefore, in the case of $P = 0.05$, the null hypothesis will be rejected *incorrectly* in 1 in 20 comparisons at this level. The *type II* error occurs when the *alternate* or *experimental* hypothesis is rejected when it is, in fact, correct. The compromise normally used to balance between type I and type II errors occurring is to set alpha at 0.05.

The notion of tailing

In concert with specifying an experimental hypothesis, a choice of statistical test will be made. In particular, it is crucial to specify whether a hypothesis is *one-tailed* or *two-tailed* because this has a major impact on the determination of the statistical test outcome. A *two-tailed* test is conducted if our hypothesis predicts a difference between two groups but does not specify the *direction* of the difference. For example, if we predict that there will be a difference in the severity of withdrawals between the FH⁺ and FH⁻ alcoholic groups but do not specify which group will express the most severe withdrawals, then we will conduct a *two-tailed test*. More realistically, of course, we would predict that the FH⁺ group would have more severe withdrawals than the FH⁻ group and therefore we would specify a *one-tailed test* because we are predetermining the direction of the difference between groups. There are important statistical considerations when deciding whether to conduct a one-tailed or a two-tailed test. By specifying the direction of the test, the one-tailed test becomes more powerful than the two-tailed test because our expectation is that the differences will be in one direction, therefore the α criterion is sensitive to just one tail of the group's score distribution. In contrast, the two-tailed test will be sensitive to both tails of the sample group's score distribution and the α criterion is spread across both tails. The upshot of all this is that for any given statistical *two-tailed* test that obtains a result with a significance level of 0.05 a *one-tailed* test would obtain a significance level 0.025. Therefore, a *two-tailed* test that obtained a result with a significance level of 0.08 would lead the researcher to conclude that there was no *statistically significant* difference between groups. However, if a *one-tailed* test had been specified, under the same conditions, the result would have a significance level of 0.04 and would, therefore, be interpreted by the researcher as evidence of a *statistically significant* difference between groups. Although the *one-tailed* test would appear to be more powerful, there is a compromise to be made in that the researcher should be quite sure that any significant differences observed will be in the direction predicted; a check on the mean scores between groups will determine whether this is the case. If a *one-tailed* test is conducted and is found to be statistically significant *but* not in the direction predicted, then the result has to be interpreted as *statistically non-significant*. Obviously, this would not be the case in the instance of a *two-tailed* test and, therefore, it is crucial that the type of test (one-tailed or two-tailed) is specified before the test is conducted. It is also obviously inappropriate to change our minds regarding the direction of predicted differences between groups after insights gained from the results of the statistical test!

Chapter 4

Study sample size calculation

Introduction

The type of experimental designs and a description of the types of data that may be encountered when conducting a clinical study have been outlined in the preceding chapters. Being satisfied that we are clear regarding our choice of IVs and DVs allows us to begin the design of the study, and a crucial aspect at this stage will be to decide the number of subjects or patients that will be required. Most often, certainly in the published literature, the number of subjects used in studies is based on a criterion that is based on convenience rather that statistical principles. This is not intended as a huge criticism because this situation is true of all disciplines and not just nursing. However, there *are* means by which sample sizes can be estimated *before* conducting a study to have a good chance of observing a statistically significant effect of IV manipulation. Put simply, this is down to the statistical truth that the more subjects per group then the more likely a statistically significant effect of the IV manipulation will be observed, all other things being equal. Therefore, it is crucial to have some kind of estimate of the *minimum* number of subjects required per group in order to observe a statistically significant IV manipulation effect. A convenient statistical procedure that is used for the calculation of minimum sample numbers is known as power analysis (Cohen, 1988). Power analysis is often applied to data gained from preliminary investigations to calculate the numbers required for a main study. However, it is not always necessary to conduct a pilot investigation to calculate minimum subject numbers if the researcher has some reasonable insight into how powerful the IV manipulation is likely to be. This is because power analysis utilises four key statistical variables, with a solution to the fourth variable readily calculated from the three other variables. These four variables are:

1. sample size (N);
2. significance level (α);
3. effect size (ES);
4. statistical power.

Therefore, when planning a study, N can be calculated from ES, α and statistical power.

Alpha (α)

As discussed in Chapter 3, α will be an arbitrary determination and will usually be taken as 0.05. A more stringent α can be set, usually at 0.01, in studies in which several hypotheses are being tested within one data set; essentially, studies in which multiple comparisons are being conducted. This makes good statistical sense of course because, where multiple comparisons are taking place, there is a greater risk of committing a type I error, and therefore setting a more stringent α such as 0.01 reduces this risk. (Multiple comparisons are discussed later in this volume.) However, for most purposes, an α criterion of 0.05 is acceptable.

Statistical power

The statistical power of a test is a function of α, ES and N and represents the probability of rejecting the null hypothesis in the long term. As the power of the test is related to probability estimations, statistical power is also subject to type II error. The probability of a type II error occurring is described as β and thus power is defined as $1 - \beta$. Fortunately, power is generally specified as a convention and is set at 0.80 (Cohen, 1988).

Effect size

The effect size can be a difficult concept for researchers to conceptualise in power analysis. However, a useful way of considering the term is to think of it as the degree to which the researcher considers the null hypothesis to be false or the alternate hypothesis to be true. The more confident that the researcher is that the IV manipulation will have a significant experimental effect, the larger the effect size would be considered to be. Quantifying this would obviously seem to be quite difficult in the absence of any prior study being conducted. Generally speaking, most researchers will design an investigation based on a thorough and systematic review of the available literature, so it is plausible for the researcher to have some idea of the probable magnitude of the IV manipulation before conducting the planned investigation. Cohen (1992) has suggested operational definitions and conventions for effect sizes termed small, medium and large. These definitions are gained from insights following Cohen's extensive review of previously published empirical research. Although it can be argued that all effect sizes are important, for example even a small effect associated with the IV manipulation of a novel drug would be of great value if it was to save just a few lives, we would argue that for most purposes, and particularly for defining the sample size of a proposed investigation, a medium effect should be specified. This is principally because, following a review of the literature, the researcher should have an expectation that their IV manipulation will have an appreciable effect on the dependent variable (DV). It would also be inappropriate to suggest that the effect size should be large during the design of a study even though the conducted study may reveal a large effect size. This is because the researcher should be using a sample size big enough to detect a medium effect size. Such a sample would also detect a large effect size. However, to detect a large effect size, smaller sample sizes can be specified, although these sample numbers would be insufficient to detect a medium effect size. We would therefore suggest that the minimum number of subjects required for a study should be based on a medium effect size, with power at 0.8 and $\alpha = 0.05$. In each of the chapters that follow, sample size estimations have been conducted for each of the experimental designs. When you begin to conduct your own studies, these will be the minimum sample sizes that you should specify for a novel investigation.

Chapter 5

Choice of statistical tests

Introduction

In the following chapters, the design and analysis of clinical studies will be explored with actual data accrued from conducted investigations. One final statistical notion has to be encountered before examination of the statistical manipulation of data within the context of the study designs so far outlined. This statistical notion relates to the *type* of statistical test.

Parametric tests

Although each type of design has an accompanying characteristic statistical test, it is important to note that, in fact, there are fundamentally only *two* types of statistical test. These two types are the *parametric* and the *non-parametric* statistical tests. The main differences between these two different test types is that the *parametric* tests make stringent assumptions regarding the type and distribution of the collected data. In contrast, the *non-parametric* tests make few assumptions about the data or the data distribution. Every simple parametric test has an equivalent non-parametric test, therefore it may seem to the novice researcher that, all things being equal, it is best to always use the non-parametric test. This is not the case because the assumptions that underpin the parametric tests make them statistically more powerful than non-parametric tests. Put simply, non-parametric tests are more conservative than parametric tests. The choice of test can therefore be crucial if the difference between two group means is on the cusp or border of statistical significance. Essentially, where the difference between two sample means is statistically borderline, the parametric test is more likely to be statistically significant than the non-parametric test. Given that parametric tests are more powerful than non-parametric tests, it is important to appraise the restrictions of the parametric test in determining which type of test will be more appropriate. There are three underlying assumptions to the use of the parametric tests, these are:

1. normal distribution;
2. interval measurement;
3. homogeneity of variance.

Normal distribution

A key parametric assumption is that the sample data are drawn from a normal population. Although it is possible to draw a histogram from the data to determine whether the data set is markedly negatively or positively skewed and to determine whether the distribution looks normal, it is actually impossible to *prove* that the data set is representative of a normal distribution. However, as the focus of the sample characteristic is the mean score (the summary statistic), it has generally been found that scores which fall around the mean in a *sample* are generally normally distributed, but *only* if there are sufficient numbers of subjects. It is more difficult to determine whether scores are normally distributed when there are only a small number of scores. Most statisticians agree that a normal distribution can be assumed in a sample size of forty or more. If there are fewer than forty subjects in the study, it is safer to assume that the normal distribution assumption is likely to be violated.

Interval measurement

A further assumption underpinning the conduct of a parametric test is that the data should be of interval or ratio measurement (discussed in Chapter 3). Ordinal and nominal scales of measurement do not satisfy the criteria for the conduct of a parametric test.

Homogeneity of variance

The parametric assumption of homogeneity of variance refers to the criteria that the compared samples should be drawn from populations with equal variance. Like the normal distribution assumption it is not possible to prove that this is indeed the case. However, it is relatively easy to detect violations to this parametric assumption. A useful rule of thumb is to compare the variance between the sample groups (remember, the variance is the square of the standard deviation). If the variance is more than four times larger between groups, then we can suggest that the sample variances between groups are *not equal* and the parametric assumption has been violated.

It would thus appear that there are many caveats to the use of parametric tests, and it may seem that it would be easier to play safe and always use non-parametric tests. Fortunately, however, statisticians have discovered that parametric tests are *very robust* even when the parametric assumptions underlying the test are violated. Accepting that it is difficult to determine that a sample has been drawn from a normal population if there are fewer than forty subjects in the study, yet it is relatively easy to determine whether samples to be compared have homogeneity of variance and it is obvious at what levels of measurement our data are, then we would suggest that it is perfectly acceptable to conduct a parametric test if the data satisfy the criteria of homogeneity of variance and interval/ ratio measurement. If fewer than two of the assumptions underlying the conduct of the parametric test are evident, then it is prudent to use the equivalent non-parametric test.

Non-parametric tests

In contrast to the parametric test assumptions outlined previously, non-parametric tests make *few* assumptions about the sample data characteristics. Most of the non-parametric tests assume only an *ordinal* level of data measurement (Chapter 3). Further, non-parametric tests make no assumptions about the population distributions either in terms of shape or variance. Non-parametric tests are therefore quite often referred to as *distribution-free* significance tests. Non-parametric tests are generally not quite as powerful as parametric tests in detecting statistically significant differences between or within groups.

An excellent overview of non-parametric statistics can be found in Siegel (1956) and Meddis (1984).

Summary

There are two types of test statistic that can be applied to research data; the first type, the parametric set of statistical tests, makes assumptions regarding the type of data and the distribution characteristics of the data. The non-parametric tests, on the other hand, make few such assumptions and can be applied in situations where the application of a parametric test would be inappropriate. The parametric tests are generally more powerful than their non-parametric counterparts. The parametric tests are also often described as robust, meaning that, even when some of the parametric assumptions underpinning the tests are violated, the tests may still, under some circumstances, be applied and accurate statistical test results obtained.

Chapter 6

Between-subjects design and tests

Introduction

The between-subjects design was described in Chapter 2. The between-subjects design, in its simplest form, compares two levels of the IV, and this represents a design format that is used as the 'gold standard' in a significant proportion of clinical research, notably clinical trials, this design being exemplified in the randomised controlled trial (RCT). In the RCT, patients are randomly allocated either to a control or to a treatment condition. In the instance of an RCT of a drug being conducted, the study design is invariably *double blind*. A 'single-blind' study is an investigation in which the patient is unaware which group they have been allocated to, either a control (placebo) group or a treatment condition group. A 'double-blind' study is an investigation in which both the patient and the investigator are unaware which group the patient has been allocated to. Blinding is a technique that is used to reduce bias in RCTs.

There are other applications of the between-subjects design in addition to the RCT. The main point is that between-subjects design uses distinctly defined groups for comparison, as outlined in Chapter 2. Although there can be any number of levels of the IV in the between-subjects design, for many purposes *two* levels are deemed adequate and appropriate. This is, of course, consistent with the notion of hypothesis testing, as most hypotheses should be able to be tested by a comparison between groups because the hypothesis focuses on the notion of a definable effect of the IV manipulation rather than such a manipulation's magnitude. Although groups may be readily defined by a diagnosis, for example a comparison between healthy controls and cancer patients, it is also possible and often desirable to define groups using an arbitrary measure which may or may not be a clinical index. We may, for example, define two groups of surgical patients based on an arbitrary criteria of age, i.e. group one < 65 years, group two ≥65 years. On the other hand, we may use a clinical index to define two groups of renal patients, group one being adequately dialysed, group two being inadequately dialysed.

A clinical example

Using the RCT design as an illustration, let us consider the following clinical question within the context of the design and statistical test type. It has been established for many years that high levels of cholesterol are implicated in the manifestation of coronary heart disease, particularly low-density lipoproteins (LDLs). A worthy research enterprise would be, therefore, to develop a medication that would reduce the level of circulating lipids, particularly in a high-risk group of patients such as those who have recently had a myocardial infarction (MI). To test whether a novel medication would be efficacious in reducing lipid levels, we would need to design a robust study and, as mentioned previously, the RCT provides the gold standard for drug evaluation studies. Ideally, we would specify our target sample, which in this case would be recent post-MI patients. These patients would then be *randomised*, i.e. randomly allocated to one of two groups, group one (control, placebo) and group two (novel drug, treatment). The study would be conducted as a *double-blind* investigation to reduce bias. In this between-subjects design, the IV would be group type (placebo/treatment) and the DV would be a measure of the expected impact of the IV manipulation; in this example, the DV would be cholesterol or lipid levels after the IV manipulation, assessed at a predetermined post-IV manipulation sampling time. Obviously, in a real-world situation, the IV could relate to a single dose of the treatment/placebo or a whole course of treatment/placebo. Assuming that the data accrued from such a study satisfied the criteria for a parametric test, the statistical test of choice within this between-subjects design would be the *between-subjects t*-test, which is often also known as the *independent* or *unrelated t*-test.

Between-subjects t-test

The mathematical formula used to compute *t* gives a measure of the size of the differences between the two groups and calculates from this a standard measure of deviation. The larger the *t*-value, the greater the differences between sample means and the *lower* the probability that the differences between group scores on the DV are a function of chance factors. If the value of *t* is great enough to reduce the probability level to 0.05 or below, then the *null hypothesis* can be rejected in favour of the *alternate* or *experimental hypothesis*. If the null hypothesis can be rejected then we can conclude that there is a statistically significant difference between the two groups and that this significant difference is due to the IV manipulation. A final important feature to consider before conducting this test is the concept of *degrees of freedom*.

Degrees of freedom

The degrees of freedom (d.f.) is a term used to describe the number of DV scores which can contribute to the DV score variance. It would initially appear that *all* subject DV scores should contribute to the variance, and this is indeed the case; however, it is also important to consider that the mean score is used in calculating the variance. It would seem then that one score from the data set, the mean score, is not free to vary because it is central to variance and standard deviation calculation. Calculation of the variance in the t-test is therefore computed on the basis of $N - 1$. As two variances are computed for the between-subjects t-test (one for each group), the t-distribution shape is dependent on the number of *freely* varying scores that are used to calculate *both* groups $(N_1 - 1)$ and $(N_2 - 1)$ or $[(N_1 + N_2) - 2]$ variances. Interpretation of t in terms of a probability value of P is consequently based on a d.f. of $(N_1 + N_2 - 2)$.

Coming back to the example stated, our two groups (control vs. treatment) DV lipid levels (mmol/l) are shown in Table 6.1. The mean score for each group is calculated using the formula described in Chapter 3.

The variance for each group is then calculated using the following formula:

Table 6.1 Control and treatment group blood lipid levels

Group I (control/placebo) (N_1 = 10) X	Group 2 (treatment) (N_2 = 10) X
5	3
3	4
5	2
5	2
7	6
6	7
8	4
6	6
5	3
6	4

$$S^2 = \frac{\sum (X - \overline{X})^2}{N - 1}$$

In this formula, the deviation of each score from the mean is calculated and then squared. The sum of the squared deviations is then divided by $N - 1$.

Calculation of the mean and variance completes the elements of data necessary to perform the t-test. These values are then substituted in the formula for t, which is as follows:

$$t = \frac{\overline{X}_1 - \overline{X}_2}{\sqrt{\left(\frac{\left((N_1 - 1) \times S_1^2\right) + \left((N_2 - 1) \times S_2^2\right)}{(N_1 + N_2 - 2)} \times \left(\frac{1}{N_1} + \frac{1}{N_2} \right) \right)}}$$

However, when the sample sizes of each group are the same, a simpler version of the t-formula is used:

$$t = \frac{\overline{X}_1 - \overline{X}_2}{\sqrt{\frac{S_1^2 + S_2^2}{N}}}$$

The example is worked out fully as follows (see Table 6.2 and the calculations immediately following).

Degrees of freedom would be calculated $(10 + 10 - 2)$. Degrees of freedom are usually stated immediately after the t and, therefore, our t value is $t(18) = 2.17$. Referring to Table A.1, t with d.f. = 18 is tabled as

Table 6.2 Individual and squared control and treatment group lipid values

Group 1 (control/placebo) (N_1 = 10)		Group 2 (treatment) (N_2 = 10)	
X_1	X_1^2	X_2	X_2^2
5	25	3	9
3	9	4	16
5	25	2	4
5	25	2	4
7	49	6	36
6	36	7	49
8	64	4	16
6	36	6	36
5	25	3	9
6	36	4	16

$\Sigma X_1 = 56$	$\Sigma X_1^2 = 330$	$\Sigma X_2 = 41$	$\Sigma X_2^2 = 195$
$\overline{X}_1 = 56/10$		$\overline{X}_2 = 41/10$	
$\overline{X}_1 = 5.60$		$\overline{X}_2 = 4.10$	

Each group variance is then calculated:

$$S_1^2 = \frac{\sum(X_1 - \overline{X}_1)^2}{N_1 - 1} \qquad\qquad S_2^2 = \frac{\sum(X_2 - \overline{X}_2)^2}{N_2 - 1}$$

$S_1^2 = 16.4/9 \qquad\qquad S_2^2 = 26.9/9$

$S_1^2 = 1.82 \qquad\qquad S_2^2 = 2.99$

Substituting these values into the t-formula:

$$t = \frac{\overline{X}_1 - \overline{X}_2}{\sqrt{\dfrac{S_1^2 + S_2^2}{N}}}$$

$$t = \frac{5.60 - 4.10}{\sqrt{\dfrac{1.82 + 2.99}{10}}}$$

$t = 1.50/0.69$

$t = 2.17$

2.101 at $\alpha = 0.05$ (two-tailed). As our calculated t-value (2.17) is greater than the tabled t-value, the alternate hypothesis is accepted and the null hypothesis is rejected. The statistical finding is reported thus: $t(18) = 2.17, P < 0.05$. The t-test revealed that there was a statistically significant difference between the two groups. Observed t has to be equal to or greater than tabled t to obtain a statistically significant difference between groups. The statistical test findings lead us to conclude that there was a significant difference between the placebo and drug conditions and, therefore, we can further conclude that, within the limitations of this experimental design, the drug was effective in reducing lipid levels.

The between-subjects t-test can be applied to any between-subjects design that satisfies the parametric assumptions to conduct the test. Where the data satisfy the parametric assumptions, the between-subjects t-test is the statistical test of choice for most RCTs.

However, it is often the case that a number of the parametric assumptions which underlie the parametric test are violated. It was made clear in Chapter 5 that the parametric tests are robust against violations to the underlying assumptions; so, quite often, investigators will use a parametric test under these circumstances, *as long* as at least one of the assumptions is supported.

The Mann–Whitney U-test

The non-parametric test that is the statistical test of choice in the between-subjects design is the Mann–Whitney *U*-test. The Mann–Whitney *U*-test makes no assumptions about the underlying population distribution and can be used on ordinal scale data. A good example of a between-subjects design that has as its dependent variable data collected on the ordinal scale is an investigation into perception of pain that has as its IV an allocation to different types of treatment groups. Often, health researchers will assess pain using a visual analogue scale (VAS) or a verbal report scale (VRS). The VAS usually consists of the presentation of a 100-mm line to the patient, who is then asked to mark by pencil or pen on the line the amount of pain they are experiencing ranging from no pain at all to extreme pain. Where the line has been marked is measured, and the patient score is indicated in mm. Although the VAS is asking the patient for a rating that is subjective (amount of pain), the score obtained on the VAS is actually *interval* rather than ordinal because the estimate of perceived pain has been translated into an index that satisfies the criteria of an interval measure (see Chapter 5). On the other hand, a VRS would ask the patient to *rank* the level of perceived pain from no pain at all to severe pain using a forced choice format with a *limited* range of pain descriptors. Typically, a VRS would be scored as such:

0 = no pain;
1 = slight pain;
2 = more than slight but less than moderate pain;
3 = moderate pain;
4 = more than moderate but less than severe pain;
5 = severe pain.

The recording of data utilising this type of scale using a limited range of descriptors *but* ranged from least to most (or vice versa) is known as using a *likert-type* scale. From a statistical point of view, it can be seen that the data are being measured using a ranking instrument and, therefore, the data are essentially of the ordinal type. The following example uses data from a study examining pain perception after general surgery. Patients have been randomly allocated to one of two groups. The IV is the type of analgesia given: either standard analgesia (group 1) or standard analgesia and Entonox in combination (group 2). Entonox is an inhalation analgesic that has not been widely used previously in the general surgery setting. The DV is the patient's score on the VRS after minor surgery. Although patients have been randomly allocated to groups, the investigation is a pilot study to determine also whether there are any unforeseen methodological problems before the operation of the main study. In the example, this has led to the situation of an unequal number of patients in each group. It is desirable that there should be equal numbers of patients in each group for most studies; unequal group subject numbers *do* occur (most often in between-groups designs), but this does not generally have a significant impact on the statistical analysis.

Mann–Whitney U-test statistical procedure

Where group sizes are unequal, the group with the fewest scores is termed N_1 and the group with the largest N_2; in the case of equal group sizes, this distinction is unimportant, although it is useful, in the case of an RCT, to allocate the N_1 term to the control group and the N_2 term to the treatment group. The combined set of scores of *both* groups is then ranked serially from the lowest to the highest value, starting with the rank number of 1. If there are ties in the scores, which there often are in likert-type score formats, the average of the rank position is taken, with each tie allocated this average ranking, but it *must* be borne in mind that this will also use up *two* rank positions. The sum of the ranks of N_1 only is calculated and called R_1. The values of N_1, N_2 and R_1 are then substituted in the following equation in order to calculate U:

$$U = N_1 N_2 + [N_1 (N_1 + 1)]/2 - R_1$$

The values of N_1, N_2 and U are then substituted in the following equation to calculate U':

$$U' = N_1 N_2 - U$$

Reference to Table A.2 indicates the critical value of U', which depends on the values of N_1 and N_2 and also on whether the hypothesis was one-tailed or two-tailed.

The example of the analgesia study is worked out fully in Table 6.3 below (and the subsequent calculation).

The choice of which value, U or U', to use to determine the critical value is based on which score is *smallest*. In the example, U is the smaller score and this value ($U = 11$) is compared with the critical value for U (Table A.2). If this value is *less than or equal to* the critical value of U, then we can reject the null hypothesis. Because the critical value of U is 3, we are again forced to concede that we have to reject the alternate hypothesis and accept the null hypothesis. The findings lead us to conclude that, *statistically*, there is no difference between the groups in terms of pain ratings and, therefore, there is no *statistically significant* difference in pain control between the control analgesia regime and the Entonox regime. Using this example, the findings would be reported as: $U = 11, P = $ n.s., $N = 11$. Reference to Table A.2 reveals that the U-value

Table 6.3 Control and treatment group pain rating scores

Group 1 (control) ($N_1 = 5$)		Group 2 (Entonox) ($N_2 = 6$)	
Score	Rank	Score	Rank
2	4.5	1	2.5
1	2.5	2	4.5
5	9.5	0	1
3	6.5	3	6.5
6	11	4	8
		5	9.5
	$R_1 = 34$		

The above values are substituted into the Mann–Whitney U-equation to calculate U and U' thus:

$$U = 5 \times 6 + [5\,(5 + 1)]/2 - 34$$

$$U = 30 + 30/2 - 34$$

$$U = 11$$

The values of N_1, N_2 and U are then substituted in the following equation to calculate U':

$$U' = 5 \times 6 - 11$$

$$U' = 30 - 11$$

$$U' = 19$$

estimation is only appropriate when there are up to a *maximum* of twenty subjects per group. When there are more than twenty subjects in one of the groups, it is still possible to conduct the Mann–Whitney test by converting U to a Z *score*. Conversion of U to a Z score is conducted by substituting values of U and N into the following formula:

$$Z = \frac{U - \frac{N_1 N_2}{2}}{\sqrt{\frac{N_1 N_2 (N_1 + N_2 + 1)}{12}}}$$

Using the above formula and assuming that we have conducted a much larger study with $N_1 = 22$ and $N_2 = 28$ and with a calculated U-value of 340, we would find:

$$Z = \frac{340 - \frac{22 \times 28}{2}}{\sqrt{\frac{22 \times 28 \times 51}{12}}}$$
$$= 0.62$$

Calculated Z is then compared with the Z-test table (Table A.3), which reports probability (P) values. The table is referenced as such: for our figure of 0.62, the 0.6 value is taken from the left-hand column and the remainder, 0.02, from the top column, and gives a probability of $P = 0.2676$ at the intersection of the two values. Therefore, it would be concluded that there is no statistically significant effect of group type and this would be reported as: $U = 340$, $Z = 0.62$, $P = $ n.s. The values given in Table A.3 are for a one-tailed test; if the hypothesis had been two-tailed, then the value of P must be doubled, i.e. for the same data that we have just analysed, but under the rubric of a two-tailed hypothesis, the P-value would be 0.5352.

Number of subjects per group

The examples illustrating the between-subjects t-test and the Mann–Whitney U-test revealed no statistically significant effects of the IV manipulation. The data sets from which the illustrative data were drawn are much larger, with a small data segment taken from each study to illustrate the mathematics of each particular test. It was mentioned in Chapter 4 that the number of subjects in each group is critical to the possibility of observing a statistically significant difference between groups. Generally, the larger the number of subjects, the more likely the possibility of observing a statistically significant difference. It is also at this point that the researcher should make some intuitive judgement regarding the size of sample that is likely to be necessary to test the proposed hypothesis and detect statistically significant differences. A pilot study may shed some light on this, or, alternatively, a review of the literature will give some indication of minimum sample sizes that would be required. However, if the researcher is conducting a truly novel study with no available or appropriate previously published research literature to suggest minimum numbers, we would make the following recommendations as minimum subject numbers for *between-subjects* designs. The following estimations are based on power calculations (Cohen, 1988) and represent minimum subject numbers. When conducting a study in which it is predicted that the IV manipulation will have a *medium effect* (see Chapter 4) on the DVs, the *minimum* number of subjects per group for a between-subjects design would be sixty-four *per group*. Therefore, where equal numbers of subjects have been allocated to each group, the minimum number of subjects required to conduct the study would be 128. When conducting a study in which it is predicted that the IV manipulation will have a *large effect* (see Chapter 4) on the DVs, the *minimum* number of subjects per group for a between-subjects design would be twenty-six *per group*. Therefore, where equal numbers of subjects have been allocated to each group, the minimum number of subjects required to conduct the study would be fifty-two.

The above estimations represent realistic *minimums* and are based on two-tailed hypotheses with $\alpha = 0.05$. Although it is statistically reasonable to assume that it is possible to manage with smaller subject numbers if the hypothesis was one-tailed, we would not recommend or advocate this; it is undoubtedly worthwhile to keep to these minimum subject requirements whether the test is one-tailed or two-tailed. It is also worth thinking about the content/power of the IV. Is it really realistic to expect a large effect or should we perhaps recruit the necessary subject numbers based on the notion that our IV manipulation is more modest, essentially a medium effect? The final basis for the decision on this point obviously lies with the experimenter, but it is almost always false economy to conduct a study in which it is fairly certain that the IV will have a medium effect but the experimenter deludes themselves into believing that the IV manipulation will have large effect *just so* the study can be conducted with a much smaller subject population. Under these circumstances, such a study is not likely to find a statistically significant difference between groups and the researcher will be left to conclude that *maybe* there is an effect somewhere, but a larger replication study will be required to test the hypothesis further. It obviously makes more sense to carry out the study with the *appropriate* number of subjects in the first place as this approach will give the researcher the best chance of finding a statistically significant effect of the IV manipulation. Researchers will generally be testing hypotheses with the hope of detecting significant differences between groups. Further, although it may not be desirable, journal reviewers are generally more impressed when confronted with statistically significant group differences than with no effect of IV manipulation, and we would have no doubt in suggesting that this is an important bias in determining whether reviewed empirical studies will be judged worthy of publication.

Chi-square test for between-subjects designs

It is readily apparent that the data collected from the clinical studies that we conduct should be as statistically rich as possible so that we can apply the more powerful parametric tests and also so that we can explore the spread and distribution of scores. It is entirely possible that the investigator may observe an unusual or inconsistent score and want to compare this individual subject with the prevailing trends in the data set. Undoubtedly, data that are scored on interval/ratio measurements have much to commend them in terms of data spread characteristics and the option to apply the more powerful parametric tests. Data scored on an ordinal level of measurement are also critically insightful in these terms because the researcher may still observe the spread of data and, indeed, as long as some of the remaining parametric assumptions are not violated a *parametric* test may still be applied under some circumstances. However, this does not mean that data measured at the nominal level of measurement provide us with few data of useful clinical importance, even though there is no mathematical mean score and data are represented by frequency counts in categories. On the contrary, nominal data can provide some of the most useful data for analysis and, within the realm of the clinical environment, have major therapeutic importance and relevance. For example, in the case of a diagnosis, a confirmation of categorical status is made; this being at an ordinal level of measurement, so an individual with a diagnosis of end-stage renal disease (ESRD) *has* the diagnosis, there is a clearly defined categorical assignment at the nominal level. A patient with ESRD may be *either* adequately or inadequately dialysed, again this is at a nominal level of measurement and represents a further categorical assignment. The categorical assignment at this level is of major clinical importance because an ESRD patient who is inadequately dialysed will be required to have a therapeutic intervention, whereas the adequately dialysed patient will continue with present treatment. Of course, the whole issue of dialysis adequacy is determined by a biological index; usually, kinetic transfer/volume urea or creatinine clearance rate, these obviously being interval/ratio levels of measurement. However, cut-off points are set on these biological measures of adequacy below which an individual is determined to be inadequately dialysed. Therefore, an interval level of measurement is transformed into a nominal level of measurement to facilitate a therapeutic intervention. We can all think of examples where this aspect of nominal measurement is critical to clinical care and clinical outcome. Taking this one step further, it has been reported that patients with ESRD may suffer from depression, but we may be interested to know whether patients who are inadequately dialysed are more depressed than patients who are adequately dialysed. Depression may also be determined by a diagnosis that is categorical and therefore represents a nominal level of measurement, i.e. depressed/non-depressed (normal). To investigate this very important and clinically relevant question, it is possible to conduct a test exploring the frequency of patients in each combination of these groups (adequately dialysed/inadequately dialysed and depressed/non-depressed) to test the hypothesis that inadequately dialysed patients are more depressed than adequately dialysed patients. This test is known as the chi-square (χ^2) test for between-subjects designs.

Frequencies are entered into a 2×2 contingency table, as shown below. The total number of patients in the study is seventy-two. Therefore, it can be seen that, in the 2×2 table (Table 6.4), there are ten patients who are *inadequately* dialysed and *not* depressed and nineteen *adequately* dialysed patients who *are* depressed.

Table 6.4 2×2 contingency table

	Inadequately dialysed	Adequately dialysed	Row total
Non-depressed	10	28	38
Depressed	15	19	34
Column total	25	47	

Table 6.5 Cell number substitution of cell frequencies

	Inadequately dialysed	Adequately dialysed	Row total
Non-depressed	C_1	C_2	$C_1 + C_2$
Depressed	C_3	C_4	$C_3 + C_4$
Column total	$C_1 + C_3$	$C_2 + C_4$	

The rationale behind this test is the fundamental assumption that the number of patients per group should be due to random allocation. The χ^2 test calculates the probability that the differences in the number of patients allocated to the groups arose as a factor of chance. The χ^2 is calculated by comparing the *expected* frequencies per group with the *actual observed* frequencies per group. As the number of patients per group is defined within the 2 × 2 contingency table, it is useful to think in terms of the number of patients per *cell* of the contingency table. The cells may be allocated cell numbers and this also allows the χ^2 computational procedure to be more easily understood. The cell frequency values may be allocated cell numbers as shown in Table 6.5.

χ^2 is then computed by substituting the values of C_1, C_2, C_3, C_4 and N into the following formula:

$$\chi^2 = \frac{N\big((C_1 C_4 - C_2 C_3) - 0.5N\big)^2}{(C_1 + C_2)(C_3 + C_4)(C_1 + C_3)(C_2 + C_4)}$$

Therefore, using the data from the renal patients:

$$\chi^2 = \frac{72\big((10 \times 19 - 28 \times 15) - 36\big)^2}{38,34,25,47}$$

$$\chi^2 = \frac{72\big((190 - 420) - 36\big)^2}{38,34,25,47}$$

(Note that in the subtraction 190 − 420 only a positive value is taken)

$$\chi^2 = \frac{72(230 - 36)^2}{38,34,25,47}$$

$$\chi^2 = \frac{72 \times 37636}{38,34,25,47}$$

$$\chi^2 = \frac{2709792}{38,34,25,47}$$

The numerator is then divided by each denominator in turn. χ^2 is therefore calculated to be 1.78. The critical value of χ^2 is calculated with reference to degrees of freedom of 1 and a two-tailed hypothesis. Although the hypothesis that was proposed regarding renal disease patients was one-tailed, the χ^2 works on the basis of the actual differences observed between groups compared with expected differences and can thus only deal with positive values. The critical value for χ^2 is 3.84 with one degree of freedom, two-tailed and a level of significance of 0.05 (Table A.4). The calculated value of χ^2 has to be equal to or greater than the critical value of 3.84 to reject the null hypothesis. As our calculated value of χ^2 is 1.78, the null hypothesis cannot be rejected and we are forced to concede that inadequately dialysed patients are *not* significantly more depressed than adequately dialysed patients.

Although the χ^2 is undeniably a useful test to examine differences between groups, it has to be accepted that the conversion of data to nominal levels loses a great deal of the power within the data set. In the above example, more of the power within the data could have been utilised by comparing the levels of depression on an interval scale measure between the adequately and inadequately dialysed groups; this would be a logical approach to the data of course as the defining measure of mood state (depressed/non-depressed) was made on the basis of the cut-off points on an interval measurement scale. There are a further number of limitations with the χ^2 test in addition to those outlined so far. First, the 2×2 contingency table covers only two-tailed tests even in the event of specifying a one-tailed experimental hypothesis, although it has been suggested that a one-tailed level can be used when there are extremely strong grounds for predicting the direction of the results. However, the 2×2 contingency table specifying a two-tailed test effectively reduces the power of the test when conducting a study using a one-tailed hypothesis. Second, and most important from an experimental rigour point of view, the χ^2 test becomes harder to interpret as the sample size decreases, and it is recommended that the χ^2 test is not used when at least one of the *expected* cell frequencies is below five. Fortunately, it is relatively easy to calculate the expected frequency for each cell by using the row and column totals at the intersection of the chosen cell. The formula for calculating the expected cell frequency is simply to multiply the row total by the column total and then to divide this figure by the total number of patients in the study. As an example, the expected frequency of C_1 in our renal patient cohort would be $38 \times 25/72 = 13.19$. On a final positive note regarding the χ^2 test, the contingency table may be extended to include more cells as long as the design remains symmetrical (i.e. 4×2, 3×3, 4×4, etc). However, the χ^2 test is invariably used within the context of a 2×2 contingency table, and this is for a very good reason: the 2×2 contingency table enables us to tell whether there is a statistically significant difference between two groups when using the χ^2 test. A larger contingency table, such as a 4×4, can tell us whether there is a statistically significant difference between groups *somewhere* within the contingency table when using the χ^2 test, but not specifically which groups are statistically different from one another. We would suggest that the χ^2 test is used in between-subjects designs only within the context of a 2×2 contingency table.

More than two levels of the independent variable in between-subjects designs

The goal of good clinical research is to keep the study design as simple as possible in order to address the research question. Two levels of the IV are usually adequate for addressing the research question in between-subjects designs and are, of course, the standard in RCTs. There may, however, be some circumstances under which three or more groups will need to be compared; under these circumstances, a different type of statistical analysis, known as one-way analysis of variance (ANOVA), is carried out. Although statistically ANOVA is related to the t-test and at its simplest represents an extension of it, there are some important methodological and interpretative considerations to explore when conducting a study with three or more groups, particularly issues relating to multiple comparisons and variations in family-wise error rate. Those readers considering conducting a study with three or more groups should refer to more specialised texts that deal with these additional issues in depth (e.g. Clark-Carter, 1997), and we would also suggest contacting a statistician for advice before proceeding.

Summary

The statistical tests in this chapter cover a variety of between-subjects design studies that have two levels of the IV. Importantly, the tests described make allowances for the type of DV data that will be collected and the type of data distribution that may be encountered in data accrued from studies conducted in the clinical area. The between-subjects t-test and the Mann–Whitney U-test are ideally suited to data that are likely to be collected under the auspices of an RCT. The χ^2 test is useful when examining group differences with respect to arbitrary diagnostic criteria and nominal data measurement, but it has a number of limitations that need to be considered by the investigator.

Chapter 7

Within-subjects design and tests

Introduction

The within-subjects design was described in Chapter 2. The within-subjects design, in common with the between-subjects design discussed in Chapter 6, in its simplest form compares two levels of the IV. However, the within-subjects design uses the same patient group and makes repeated observations on this group. Therefore, the patient can act as their own control condition in terms of an experimental manipulation. The within-subjects design is often used to compare changes in a cohort of patients over time, usually in response to a therapeutic intervention or to examine changes in the patient in response to treatment stage or disease state. The within-subjects design is perhaps the most robust experimental design because it intrinsically controls for individual patient's characteristics by using the same group of patients.

A clinical example

Following on from the example of post-MI patients in Chapter 6, it is worth considering some further data collected on this patient group at the time of admission and on *day 5* of admission. We would therefore be using the within-subjects design because we are going to measure a DV at two distinct time intervals, but within the *same group* of patients. In this example, our IV is the time of DV observation, of which there are two levels, at time of admission and day 5 after admission. The DV in this instance is self-report anxiety status using a brief questionnaire. The issue of anxiety is becoming increasingly important in cardiac research as it has become linked with outcome after MI (Martin and Thompson, 2000a; Martin *et al.*, 2000). There is, therefore, an entirely justifiable and valid reason to investigate the issue of anxiety within this clinical population. The cardiac example in Chapter 6 used a biological DV; in this example, we are going to use a psychological DV. The types of design discussed in this volume apply just as readily to biological and psychological variables and would therefore cover most of the types of data that the nurse researcher would be likely to encounter when conducting quantitative nursing research. We have therefore once again specified our target sample, which is recent post-MI patients. We have also specified the levels of the IV (time of admission/5 days after admission) and the nature of our DV (self-report anxiety). Obviously, in this instance, it is quite impractical, and indeed inappropriate, to conduct a double-blind study because it is fairly obvious that the data collection instrument is an index of affective status and we would not of course be randomising patients to groups as we are intending to use one group of patients under *all* IV conditions.

Assuming that the data accrued from such a study satisfied the criteria for a parametric test, the statistical test of choice for this within-subjects design would be the *within-subjects* *t*-test, which is often also known as the *related* *t*-test. The within-subjects *t*-test is the most powerful test statistically speaking for analysing within-subject experimental designs.

Within-subjects *t*-test

In common with the between-subjects *t*-test discussed in the previous chapter, the mathematical formula used to compute *t* in the within-subjects *t*-test gives a measure of the size of the differences between the two groups and calculates from this a standard measure of deviation. The larger the *t*-value, the greater the differences between sample means and the *lower* the probability that the differences between group scores on the DV are a function of chance factors. If the value of *t* is great enough to reduce the probability level to 0.05 or below, then the *null hypothesis* can be rejected in favour of the *alternate* or *experimental hypothesis*. If the null hypothesis can be rejected then we can conclude that there is a statistically significant difference between the DV measures as a function of the IV manipulation. The concept of *degrees of freedom* is of central importance to the within-subjects *t*-test and has been discussed in the previous chapter at length.

Coming back to the example outlined, the self-report anxiety ratings of the cohort of post-MI patients on admission and on day 5 after admission are shown in Table 7.1. The index of anxiety used measures anxiety on an ascending scale, therefore higher scores are associated with relatively greater anxiety.

Table 7.1 Post-MI self-report anxiety scores

Patient number	On admission (X_1)	Day 5 of admission (X_2)
1	5	3
2	3	3
3	5	4
4	5	2
5	4	3
6	11	2
7	11	8
8	11	3
9	6	2
10	9	4

A difference score (d) between the two DV scores is calculated ($X_1 - X_2$) and this is then followed by the calculation of the square of d (d^2) (see Table 7.2). The sum of d (Σd) and d^2 (Σd^2) is then calculated: $\Sigma d = 36$, $\Sigma d^2 = 210$.

The mean of d (dm) is then calculated: $\Sigma d / N = 36/10$, therefore $dm = 3.60$. The standard deviation of the differences (SD_d) is then calculated by substitution of the observed values into the following formula:

$$SD_d = \sqrt{\frac{\sum d^2}{N} - dm^2}$$

Therefore:

Table 7.2 Post-MI self-report anxiety difference scores

Patient number	On admission (X_1)	Day 5 of admission (X_2)	d $(X_1 - X_2)$	d^2
1	5	3	2	4
2	3	3	0	0
3	5	4	1	1
4	5	2	3	9
5	4	3	1	1
6	11	2	9	81
7	11	8	3	9
8	11	3	8	64
9	6	2	4	16
10	9	4	5	25

$$SD_d = \sqrt{\frac{210}{10} - (3.60)^2}$$
$$= \sqrt{21 - 12.96}$$
$$= \sqrt{8.05}$$
$$= 2.84$$

The value of t is then calculated by substituting the value obtained above into the following formula:

$$t = \frac{dm}{SD_d / \sqrt{N-1}}$$

Therefore:

$$t = \frac{3.60}{2.84 / \sqrt{9}}$$
$$= 3.60/0.94$$
$$= 3.82$$

The critical value of t is then found with reference to Table A.1 for a significance level of 0.05. The critical value is dependent on the degrees of freedom ($N - 1$) and whether the hypothesis was one-tailed or two-tailed. If the observed t (3.82) is equal to or greater than tabled t then the null hypothesis can be rejected in favour of the alternate hypothesis. Referring to Table A.1, tabled t with nine degrees of freedom is 2.26 (two-tailed); as observed t is greater than tabled t then we can conclude that there is a statistically significant difference between anxiety levels taken on the day of admission and on day 5 and conclude that anxiety decreases significantly over a 5-day period after MI (alternate hypothesis). This result would be reported as $t(9) = 3.82, P < 0.05$.

The within-subjects t-test is extremely useful and, as stated earlier, is the most powerful statistical test for within-subjects designs. Because the within-subjects t-test is a parametric test, it is important that the parametric assumptions underlying the test should not be extensively violated so that the use of the within-subjects t-test is not compromised or invalidated (see Chapter 5). There is, however, a non-parametric test that can be used for within-subjects designs that makes no assumptions about population distributions, this is the *Wilcoxon* test.

Wilcoxon test

The Wilcoxon test, also known and described more comprehensively as the Wilcoxon matched pairs signed ranks statistical test, is an extremely useful test for analysing within-subjects designs. The Wilcoxon test is the non-parametric equivalent of the within-subjects *t*-test and makes no assumptions about normal distributions. The Wilcoxon test can be readily applied to both ordinal and interval levels of measurement. Interestingly, although the Wilcoxon test is not statistically as powerful as the within-subjects *t*-test, it is *nearly* as powerful as the within-subjects *t*-test and is indeed the most powerful *non-parametric* test for the analysis of within-subjects designs. The Wilcoxon test is also by far the most widely used non-parametric test for within-subjects designs. The principal requirement needed to satisfy the criteria to conduct the Wilcoxon test is that the data can be *ranked* in ascending order. The Wilcoxon test procedure takes into account the possibility of tied scores, although an increasing number of tied scores reduces the statistical power of the test a little; however, taking into account the characteristics of most data sets that can be ranked, this small loss of statistical power is of little consequence and the test remains valid and appropriate in most circumstances. To illustrate the Wilcoxon test, we shall once again use an example drawn from clinical data.

Clinical example: alcohol dependency and depression

There is a great deal of research literature that suggests that alcohol dependency is associated with a constellation of psychopathology, including depression (Otter and Martin, 1996). Indeed, a diagnosis of alcohol dependency, alcohol abuse or alcoholism is often made within the context of a dual diagnosis that may include depression. Typically, alcohol-dependent individuals are generally more depressed than non-alcoholic individuals and extensive use of psychopharmacotherapy is used to treat such individuals, most often in the form of antidepressant medication. The following example data are drawn from a representative subset of alcohol-dependent individuals participating in a study which investigated the possibility that increasing the amount of carbohydrate in the diet would result in a decrease in depression in alcohol-dependent individuals. The rationale for this is that increasing the amount of carbohydrate in the diet increases the amount of the neurotransmitter serotonin in the brain; reduced levels of serotonin have been associated with depression and alcohol dependency (Martin and Bonner, 2000).

Subjects were assessed on two occasions (on two separate days) 2.5 hours after being given on one occasion a nutritionally balanced breakfast and on the other occasion a breakfast high in carbohydrates. The IV is therefore breakfast type (nutritionally balanced or high in carbohydrates), and the DV is self-report depression score on a standard twenty-one-item depression index. Because this is a within-subjects design, the participants will, in fact, have each breakfast on two separate occasions. However, we may be concerned that the participants may respond differently to the questionnaire on its second administration as a result of being familiar with it after its first administration. This possibility of experimental confound is known as an *order effect*. There is, however, a way for controlling for this and that is to ensure that half of the participants have the nutritionally balanced, or control, breakfast on the first occasion and the remaining participants have the high carbohydrate breakfast on the first occasion. The participants would then be *crossed over* to the other breakfast condition for the second occasion. By *counterbalancing* the study in this way, we are taking into account the possibility that the participants may respond slightly differently to the questionnaire on the second administration. However, we can be sure that if a significant difference is observed in depression scores as a function of the IV manipulation then this is down to the IV manipulation itself and *not* an order effect. Because we shall assume that the data are from an exploratory study, with no prior research being conducted in this area regarding dietary manipulation, we shall specify a two-tailed hypothesis; essentially, we predict that there will be a difference between conditions as a result of the IV manipulation *but we will not* specify the expected direction of the difference. This is a useful approach to adopt in exploratory studies as it is entirely possible that IV manipulation *does indeed* have a significant effect but via a different biological mechanism than we anticipate, and therefore it is entirely feasible that the result may be in a counterintuitive direction (see Chapter 3 for more on this point and rationale). The data are shown in Table 7.3. In this example, higher scores relate to higher levels of depression.

The initial computation in the Wilcoxon test is to calculate d, between the DV score pairs $(X_1 - X_2)$. This is the same as we saw with the MI data previously using the within-subjects t-test; negative values should be recorded. Then the d scores are *ranked* from lowest to highest, at this stage positive and negative weightings to the d scores are *ignored* in the ranking process. Although the smallest values are given the rank rating of 1, special account has to be given for *ties*. There are *two* types of possible ties: these are ties *between score pairs* and ties *between d scores*.

Table 7.3 Self-report depression scores as a function of breakfast type

Patient number	Control breakfast (X_1)	High-carbohydrate breakfast (X_2)
1	19	17
2	8	4
3	18	22
4	30	22
5	23	20
6	22	20
7	20	20
8	12	18
9	19	15
10	13	3

In the instance of a tie between score pairs and therefore $d = 0$, the score pair in question is omitted and the value of N is reduced to reflect this. In the case of two or more d scores being tied, each d score is given the average score of the ranks that would have been used should there not have been a tie between d scores. The calculation of these values with respect to the data set discussed is illustrated in Table 7.4.

The ranks of the *least* occurring sign (positive or negative) are then summed and given a value T. In this example set, there are only two negative values (−4 and −6), and therefore the corresponding rank values are summed. T therefore is $5 + 7 = 12$. The critical value of T for 0.05 significance is found with reference to Table A.5. The critical value is dependent on the value of N and whether the hypothesis was one-tailed or two-tailed. If observed T is less than or equal to tabled T then the null hypothesis may be rejected in favour of the alternate hypothesis. In the example, tabled T for $N = 9$ (remember one score pair was omitted as a tie) and for a two-tailed hypothesis is 6. As our observed was greater

Table 7.4 Self-report depression score ranking procedure

Patient number	Control breakfast (X_1)	High-carbohydrate breakfast (X_2)	$(X_1 - X_2)$	Rank d
1	19	17	2	1.5
2	8	4	4	5
3	18	22	−4	5
4	30	22	8	8
5	23	20	3	3
6	22	20	2	1.5
7	20	20	0	Excluded
8	12	18	−6	7
9	19	15	4	5
10	13	3	10	9

than that tabled, we are forced to accept the null hypothesis and reject the alternate hypothesis, i.e. there is no statistically significant difference between conditions as a result of the IV manipulation and therefore there is no evidence from our study that dietary manipulation has an impact on self-report depression. This result would be reported as $T = 12$, $P =$ n.s., two-tailed, $N = 9$. T-values can be calculated for up to twenty-five subjects. When there are more than twenty-five subjects in the study, a Z score is required to be calculated. This is similar to what we have seen earlier in Chapter 6 in relation to the Mann–Whitney U-test. However, calculation of the Z score is slightly different and is shown by substitution of the appropriate values in the following formula:

$$Z = \frac{T - \dfrac{N(N-1))}{4}}{\sqrt{\dfrac{N(N+1)(2N+1)}{24}}}$$

The critical value for Z will be found in Table A.3, and observed Z is compared with tabled Z in exactly the same way as was shown for the Mann–Whitney U-test in Chapter 6. It is worth noting that the above formula often calculates an observed Z-value which is negative; however. this in no way affects the interpretation of the result.

Number of subjects per group

The examples illustrating the within-subjects t-test and the Wilcoxon test revealed some interesting findings. A statistically significant effect of the IV manipulation was observed in the case of MI patients' anxiety between the two time points, whereas no statistically significant effect of IV manipulation was found with regard to dietary effect on level of depression in alcohol-dependent individuals. This should not really be too much of a surprise. It is widely reported that MI patients experience greatly elevated anxiety after infarction and that this level decreases rapidly over the days following admission to the coronary care unit. The role of dietary factors in mood state and depression status has been researched far less and, indeed, is a novel area of research endeavour generally. It can, therefore, come as no surprise that there was no significant effect of dietary manipulation, particularly as the example data set used for illustrative purposes comprised only ten participants. In common with the data presented in Chapter 6, the data sets from which the illustrative data were drawn are much larger, with a small data segment taken from each study to illustrate the mathematics of each particular test. It has been mentioned in previous chapters that the larger the number of subjects the more likely the possibility of observing a statistically significant difference. The point has also been made that the researcher should make some intuitive judgement regarding the size of sample that is likely to be necessary to test the proposed hypothesis and detect statistically significant differences (see Chapters 3 and 4). A pilot study may shed some light on this, or, alternatively, a review of the literature will give some indication of minimum sample sizes that would be required. Assuming the researcher is conducting a truly novel study with no available or appropriate previously published research literature to suggest minimum numbers, we would make the following recommendations as minimum subject numbers for *within-subjects* designs. The following estimations are based on power calculations (Cohen, 1988) and represent minimum subject numbers. When conducting a study in which it is predicted that the IV manipulation will have a *medium effect* (see Chapter 4) on the DVs, the *minimum* number of subjects required for a within-subjects design would be thirty-five in total. When conducting a study in which it is predicted that the IV manipulation will have a *large effect* (see Chapter 4) on the DVs, the *minimum* number of subjects required for a within-subjects design would be fifteen in total. These estimations represent realistic *minimums* and are based on two-tailed hypotheses with $\alpha = 0.05$. We would advocate strongly that these subject numbers represent absolute *minimums* irrespective of whether the hypothesis is two-tailed or one-tailed. It may be seen with reference to Chapter 4 that it is possible to conduct within-subjects design studies with far smaller subject numbers than are required for between-subjects designs. This is largely because of the benefits of within-subjects designs, which use the same subjects under all the conditions of the IV manipulation and therefore reduce variability due to individual differences. The within-subjects design may therefore be extremely useful, particularly if there are limitations in the number of available participants or patients prepared, or able, to take part in the proposed investigation.

More than two levels of the independent variable in within-subjects designs

The goal of good clinical research is to keep the study design as simple as possible in order to address the research question, as has been stated throughout this volume. In keeping with the recommendations in the last chapter regarding between-subjects designs, two levels of the IV are usually adequate for addressing the research question in within-subjects designs. On rare occasions where circumstances dictate that three or more levels of the IV are required to address the research question, a different type of statistical analysis is carried out that is known as one-way analysis of variance (ANOVA). Although statistically ANOVA is related to the t-test and at its most simple represents an extension of it, there are some important methodological and interpretative considerations to explore when conducting a study with three or more levels of the IV, particularly issues relating to multiple comparisons and variations in family-wise error rate. Those readers considering conducting a study with three or more levels of the IV should refer to more specialised texts that deal with these additional issues in depth (e.g. Clark-Carter, 1997), and we would also suggest contacting a statistician for advice before proceeding.

Summary

The statistical tests in this chapter cover the two main within-subjects design studies that have two levels of the IV. The tests described make allowances for the type of DV data collected and the type of data distribution that may be encountered in data accrued from studies conducted in the clinical area. The within-subjects t-test is the most powerful statistical test for analysing within-subject designs described so far, although it is a parametric test and makes assumptions regarding data distribution and level of measurement. The non-parametric Wilcoxon test makes no assumptions about the distribution of the data, the only criteria for this test is that the data can be ranked. The Wilcoxon test is extremely useful because it can be used with data measured at the ordinal level of measurement and the test is *nearly* as powerful as the within-subjects t-test. It has also become clear that, compared with between-subjects designs, within-subjects designs are much more economical in terms of participant number requirements.

Chapter 8

Mixed-group design and tests

Introduction

The relative merits of between-subjects design and within-subjects design studies have been discussed in Chapters 6 and 7. It is fair to say that, where experimental manipulation of an IV is concerned, the between-subjects and within-subjects designs cover most circumstances that the researcher is likely to be confronted with when needing to conduct and design a study. However, there are occasions when it is desirable to combine the features of the between-subjects and within-subjects designs and carry out the appropriate statistical test. Chapter 3 gave an example of this in the case of examining the severity of withdrawal symptoms over time (within-subjects aspect) in two groups of alcoholics, those with a family history of alcoholism (FH$^+$) and those without a family history of alcoholism (FH$^-$) (between-subjects aspect). There are other circumstances in which a mixed design may be appropriate, for example examining the effect of sex (between-subjects aspect) on the course of malignant disease between time of diagnosis and at 6-month follow-up (within-subjects aspect). At the simplest level, the mixed-group design consists of the manipulation of two IVs, one of which is a between-subjects IV and the other a within-subjects IV. The DV, of course, remains the same in terms of quality and as described in preceding chapters.

The notion of interaction

One aspect which makes mixed-group designs particularly powerful is that they produce, even at the most basic mixed-group design type, *three levels* of results. The first two levels are known as *main effects* and represent the results of the manipulation of each IV, irrespective of the remaining IV. Therefore, within the context of the mixed-group design, the first level would give the main effect of the between-subjects aspect and the second level would give the main effect of the within-subjects aspect. In many ways, this is similar to conducting a between-subjects *t*-test and a within-subjects *t*-test, although the mathematics involved in the test procedure is of course more sophisticated than those tests that were covered in Chapters 6 and 7. However, the results of both main effects will give us a finding that we can interpret as being either statistically significant or not, as the case may be. The *third* level of results is in many ways the most interesting in the mixed-group data analysis and is known as the *interaction* effect. The interaction is the most important result in terms of interpretation and, for this reason, is often known and referred to as the *higher order interaction*. A simple definition of an interaction is where one IV is affected by another IV; therefore, there is an interaction effect. An example of an interaction is illustrated in Figure 8.1 with respect to FH⁺ and FH⁻ alcohol-dependent individuals during detoxification.

It is clear to see that at the beginning of detoxification (day 1) there is little difference between the FH⁺ and FH⁻ alcoholics in terms of the severity of withdrawals; however, later in the detoxification (day 3), there is a much larger difference in the severity of withdrawals between the FH⁺ and FH⁻ groups. It is clear that FH status (between-subjects IV) has a different impact on the severity of withdrawals at different levels of detoxification (within-subjects IV). The result will inform us as to whether this is a statistically significant interaction or not.

There are some important points to be aware of when interpreting interactions. First, it is possible to have a statistically significant interaction between both IVs *in the absence* of any statistically significant

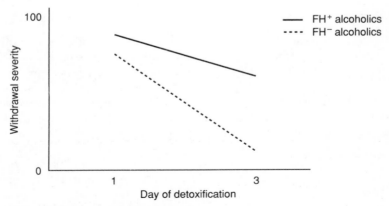

Figure 8.1 Interaction of group by time

main effects of each IV. Second, if there is found to be a statistically significant interaction, this is *always* the most important result to report on even in the *presence* of IV main effects. Third, if there is a *non-statistically significant* trend towards an interaction, an *interaction effect* should not be reported; it is important under these circumstances to report that no interaction was observed between the IVs.

Obviously, the interaction term brings a whole new level of sophistication and interpretative power to the mixed-group design and the data set to be analysed in general. However, before getting carried away and deciding that the mixed design study is the most appropriate because of these characteristics, it is vitally important to be sure that after review of the literature and formulation of an experimental hypothesis, or hypotheses, the mixed-groups design is indeed the most appropriate. This is because we must be confident that we are predicting an interaction and that this is vital to addressing the research question and we are therefore justified in using the mixed-group design; if, under these circumstances, a significant interaction is observed, this is all well and good. However, consider an alternative possibility; suppose we have not really thought out our hypothesis clearly and that this hypothesis does not really predict an interaction but just main effects. In the instance of *this study* revealing a significant interaction term, we could find ourselves in great difficulty explaining this in relation to the experimental hypothesis even if we observe our desired statistically significant main effects simply because the significant interaction is the most important finding and its observation takes precedence over any statistically significant main effects that may have been observed.

Analysis of variance

It was mentioned earlier in this chapter that the statistical method of analysing mixed-group design is mathematically similar to the between-groups and within-groups *t*-tests. The statistical test procedure for analysing mixed-group designs is known as *analysis of variance* and is often abbreviated to the term ANOVA. There are a number of methods of conducting ANOVA that are contextually sensitive to the specified experimental design type, however, the most important preliminary point to be aware of when using ANOVA is that this is a *parametric* test procedure. Therefore, the use of ANOVA is underpinned by the same parametric assumptions and rationale that are appropriate to conducting the between-subjects and within-subjects *t*-test; this of course also includes limitations and restrictions (see Chapter 5 for a résumé of these).

A clinical example

To illustrate the mixed-group design, we will draw upon further data accrued from the study on anxiety following MI that was outlined in Chapter 7. This was a study which showed that there was a significant decrease in anxiety between admission time and day 5 after admission following MI and was described in the context of a within-subjects design. We will now take some further data from that study and extend this to the context of the mixed-group design. Remember from Chapter 7 that our within-subjects IV was the time of DV observation, of which there are two levels: at time of admission and at day 5 after admission. The DV in this instance was self-report anxiety status using a brief questionnaire. It was stated that the issue of anxiety is becoming increasingly important in cardiac research as it has become linked with mortality after MI (Martin and Thompson, 2000a). This gave us an entirely justifiable and valid reason to investigate the issue of anxiety within this particular clinical population. Further, we may wish to consider other possible risk factors that may contribute to outcome and mortality after MI, and these could quite reasonably be important between-subjects variables such as age or sex. There is some evidence to suggest that women experience greater levels of anxiety after MI than men (Uuskula, 1996). This is potentially a very important phenomenon to investigate because a sex-related difference in anxiety after MI may be of great value in the design of optimal rehabilitation packages for individuals after MI. As this sex difference in anxiety is likely to relate to a cognitive component of anxiety (Martin and Thompson, 2000a), it is likely that a sex-related difference in anxiety after MI will be observed some time following the infarct rather than *immediately* after the onset of MI. Therefore, we have added a between-subjects IV (sex) with two levels (male/female) to the within-subjects design discussed in Chapter 7 and created a mixed-group design with two IVs but the same DV (self-report anxiety). As there are two levels of each IV, this type of design is often referred to as a 2 × 2 mixed-group design. For the purposes of clarity, it is useful to include the IV characteristics in the design description; so, in the instance of the study outlined, it could be described as a 2 (sex) × 2 (observation time) mixed-group design with observation time as the within-subjects factor.

Having circumscribed the experimental design and investigated the literature, we would have formulated some experimental hypotheses. First, we would predict that there will be a significant main effect of observation time (within-subjects IV) with a statistically significant decrease in anxiety at the second observation compared with the first.

Second, and more importantly, we would also predict a statistically significant interaction between sex (between-subjects IV) and observation time (within-subjects IV), and we would specifically expect there to be little difference in anxiety between sexes on admission after MI but expect women to be significantly more anxious than men on day 5 after admission. It is fairly clear that the hypothesis relating to the predicted interaction effect is of far greater clinical interest than the first hypothesis that predicts the readily established reduction in anxiety after MI over time.

Calculation of the 2 × 2 mixed-group ANOVA

For illustrative purposes, we have taken a subset of data from a larger study. The data are drawn from ten patients, five of whom are male and the remaining five of whom are female. The data are shown in Table 8.1 for all ten patients. It is clear from the layout of the data that the study is defined by two IVs: sex (between subjects) and observation time (within subjects).

To conduct the ANOVA, it is necessary to calculate the between-subjects variance and the within-subjects variance. Further, an additional statistical term called *sums of squares* will need to be calculated. This new term need not cause undue distress as it is simply a shortened description of the sum of squared deviations and is thus directly related to variance discussed in Chapter 3. In conducting the ANOVA, we will therefore have to calculate the between-subjects sums of squares and the within-subjects sums of squares (SS). First, the mean score for all *combinations* of DV defined by both IVs will need to be calculated. Further, an individual

Table 8.1 Anxiety score as a function of gender and admission time

Patient number	On admission (X_1)	Day 5 of admission (X_2)
Male patients		
1	3	0
2	6	2
3	4	1
4	1	2
5	3	2
Female patients		
6	7	3
7	5	2
8	9	3
9	2	0
10	6	2

mean score is required to be calculated for each patient across the within-subjects condition. This all sounds complicated but is, in fact, very simple and is illustrated in Table 8.2.

The overall standard deviation must then be calculated (SD = 2.37), as must the overall variance term (SD^2 = 5.61). Once these terms are known, the total SS (SS_{Total}) is then calculated using the following formula:

SS_{Total} = $SD^2 \times N - 1$ (which in this case is the N of scores)

Therefore, $5.61 \times 19 = 106.59$

SS_{Total} =   106.59

Having calculated the SS_{Total}, the between-subjects SS is then calculated by calculating the mean score for each patient and then calculating the sum of the squared deviations from the overall mean for these means. The squared deviation is then multiplied by the number of scores contributing to each patient's mean, which in this case would be a factor of 2. The calculated figure is then summed to give the between-subjects SS. The process of calculating the between-subjects SS is shown in Table 8.3. The between-subjects SS is thus calculated to be 48.05.

Table 8.2 Anxiety score as a function of gender and admission time mean score calculation

Patient number	On admission (X_1)	Day 5 of admission (X_2)	Sex mean	Patient mean
Male patients				
1	3	0		1.5
2	6	2		4
3	4	1		2.5
4	1	2		1.5
5	3	2		2.5
Mean	3.4	1.4	2.4	
Female patients				
6	7	3		5
7	5	2		3.5
8	9	3		6
9	2	0		1
10	6	2		4
Mean	5.8	2	3.9	
Time mean	4.6	1.7		

Notes
Overall mean = (3.4 + 1.4 + 5.8 + 2)/4 = 3.15

Table 8.3 Anxiety score as a function of gender and admission time deviation calculation

Patient number	Patient mean	Deviation from overall mean (3.15)	Deviation squared	Deviation squared × 2
Male patients				
1	1.5	−1.65	2.72	5.44
2	4	0.85	0.72	1.45
3	2.5	−0.65	0.42	0.84
4	1.5	−1.65	2.72	5.44
5	2.5	−0.65	0.42	0.84
Female patients				
6	5	1.85	3.42	6.85
7	3.5	0.35	0.12	0.25
8	6	2.85	8.12	16.25
9	1	−2.15	4.62	9.25
10	4	0.85	0.72	1.45

The between-subjects SS for the between-subjects IV (sex) is then found by calculating the sum of the squared deviations of the mean score for *each sex* irrespective of the observation time condition. The solution to between-subjects IV (sex) SS also termed SS_A is almost identical to the solution for calculating the total SS. The calculated figure is then summed to give the between-subjects IV SS_A and is illustrated in Table 8.4.

The between-subjects IV SS_A is thus calculated to be 11.2.

A subjects within groups SS $[SS_{S(groups)}]$ must now be calculated and is simply the between-subjects SS minus SS_A. Therefore:

$$SS_{S(groups)} = 48.05 - 11.2$$
$$SS_{S(groups)} = 36.85$$

The SS for the within-subjects IV (SS_B) observation time is then calculated: the sum of the squared deviations of the mean score for *each observation time* irrespective of the sex condition. The solution is almost identical to the solution for calculating the total SS. The calculated figure

Table 8.4 Between-subjects component calculation

Sex	Patient mean	Deviation from overall mean (3.15)	Deviation squared	Deviation squared × 2
Male	2.4	−0.75	0.56	5.6
Female	3.9	0.75	0.56	5.6

Table 8.5 Within-subjects component calculation

Time	Patient mean	Deviation from overall mean (3.15)	Deviation squared	Deviation squared × 10
Day 1	4.6	1.45	2.1	21
Day 5	1.7	−1.45	2.1	21

is then summed to give the within-subjects IV SS_B and is illustrated in Table 8.5. The within-subjects IV SS_B is thus calculated to be 42.

The interaction (sex × time) SS is then calculated; this term is defined as SS_{AB}. This is found by initially obtaining the means for the sex × time cells and calculating the SS term, as we have seen previously, this is illustrated in Table 8.6.

The SS of the between-subjects IV × the within-subjects IV is 57.35. The interaction term SS_{AB} is then calculated by subtracting the sum of SS_A and SS_B from the SS of the between-subjects IV × the within-subjects IV, thus:

$$SS_{AB} = 57.35 - (11.2 + 42)$$

$$SS_{AB} = 4.15$$

Finally, the within-subjects IV within groups SS [$SS_{B \text{ by } S(groups)}$] is calculated. This obtained as follows:

$$SS_{B \text{ by } S(groups)} = SS_{Total} - [SS_A + SS_{S(groups)} + SS_B + SS_{AB}]$$

$$SS_{B \text{ by } S(groups)} = 106.59 - (11.2 + 36.85 + 42 + 4.15)$$

$$SS_{B \text{ by } S(groups)} = 106.59 - 94.2$$

$$SS_{B \text{ by } S(groups)} = 12.39$$

Table 8.6 Interaction component calculation

Sex	Patient mean	Deviation from overall mean (3.15)	Deviation squared	Deviation squared × 5
Male				
Day 1	3.4	0.25	0.6	0.31
Day 5	1.4	−1.75	3.06	15.31
Female				
Day 1	5.8	2.65	7.02	35.11
Day 5	2.0	−1.15	1.32	6.61

Calculation of the degrees of freedom for mixed-group ANOVA

Between subjects

The between-subjects degrees of freedom (d.f.) is calculated as $2 - 1 = 1$. The subjects within group d.f. is calculated on the basis that *each* group's d.f. $= 5 - 1 = 4$. As there are two groups, the subjects within groups d.f. is equal to 8.

Within subjects

The within-subjects d.f. is calculated as observation time d.f. $= 2 - 1 = 1$. The interaction between sex and time $= 1 \times 1 = 1$. Finally, the sex by time within group $= 1 \times 8 = 8$.

A summary table is then produced from the accrued data to calculate a *mean square* and an *F-value*. The mean square term is simply the relevant SS divided by the appropriate degrees of freedom. The *F*-value is calculated by dividing the appropriate IV mean squares by either the $SS_{S(groups)}$ or the $SS_{B \text{ by } S(groups)}$ mean square term. The summary table (Table 8.7) illustrates the final calculations involved in solving for the *F*-value.

The *F*-value obtained for each level of the ANOVA is then compared with tabled values (Table A.6) to determine statistical significance at the 0.05 level. Tabled *F* is determined by the intersection of the IV d.f. and the group, also known as variance *error* term d.f. In Table A.6, the IV d.f. is read from the top of the table and error term is read from the side. In the case of the study outlined, tabled *F*-value for an IV d.f. of 1 and an error term of 8 is found to be 5.32. The observed *F*-value should be equal to or greater than tabled *F* in order to conclude that there is a statistically significant effect of the IV manipulation. Interpreting the results, we are forced to concede that there is no statistically significant main effect of sex, and this would be described in the following way: $F(1,8) = 2.45$, $P =$ n.s. It can be seen that the d.f. for the IV and the error term are included directly after the *F* statement. A statistically significant effect of observation time was observed, however, revealing a significant

Table 8.7 ANOVA summary table

Variance source	d.f.	Sum of squares	Mean square	F-value
IV sex	1	11.2	11.2	2.45
Subject (group)	8	36.85	4.61	
IV time	1	42	42	27.10
IV time by sex	1	4.15	4.15	2.68
Time by sex (group)	8	12.39	1.55	

reduction in anxiety between that observed on admission and on day 5 after admission: $F(1,8) = 27.10$, $P < 0.05$. Contrary to the stated experimental hypothesis, there was no evidence of a statistically significant interaction between sex and observation time: $F(1,8) = 2.68$, $P = $ n.s. We are therefore forced to concede that our data did not support our hypothesis regarding sex on perceived levels of patient anxiety after MI.

Non-parametric tests for mixed-group designs

Invariably, the most widely used statistical test for analysing mixed-group designs is the parametric ANOVA. Often, researchers will use ANOVA when one or more of the parametric assumptions required to conduct this parametric test are violated, justifying this by using the rationale that the test procedure itself is very robust against such violations (Chapter 5). Additionally, computer statistical packages tend to have exclusively only parametric tests available for mixed-group design analysis and therefore non-parametric equivalent tests are underrepresented in this respect. We would suggest that, in the case of the mixed-group design, ANOVA can be appropriate for data sets that do not support all the parametric assumptions *so long as* the data are *at least* of the ordinal level of measurement or greater. There are some specialist texts which deal with the analysis of mixed-group designs using non-parametric test criteria and the interested reader should refer to this for further details and the required formulae (Meddis, 1984).

Number of subjects per group

In the absence of pilot data or previously published research papers, the researcher will be required to justify the minimum number of subjects required to conduct the study in order to have a realistic chance of finding some statistically significant differences somewhere within the data set. It has been emphasised a number of times in this volume that the researcher should make some intuitive judgement regarding the size of sample that is likely to be necessary to test the proposed hypothesis and detect statistically significant differences (see Chapters 4 and 5). Should the researcher be conducting a truly novel study with no available or appropriate previously published research literature to suggest minimum numbers, we would make the following recommendations as minimum subject numbers for *mixed-group* designs. Consistent with sample size estimations from previous chapters, the following estimations are based on power calculations (Cohen, 1988) and represent minimum subject numbers. When conducting a study in which it is predicted that the IV manipulation will have a *medium effect* (see Chapter 4) on the DVs, the *minimum* number of subjects required for a mixed-group design would be 140 in total. When conducting a study in which it is predicted that the IV manipulation will have a *large effect* (see Chapter 4) on the DVs, the *minimum* number of subjects required for a mixed-group design would be sixty in total. These estimations represent realistic *minimums* and are based on a probability $\alpha = 0.05$. We would advocate strongly that these subject numbers represent absolute *minimums* irrespective of whether the hypothesis is two-tailed or one-tailed.

More than two levels of each independent variable in the mixed-group design

Although the 2×2 mixed group ANOVA represents the most widely used and simplest mixed-group design, it is possible to conduct a mixed-group study with IVs with three or more levels. It is also possible to conduct a mixed-group study with more than two IVs. We would suggest that, and consistent with our recommendations on the between-subjects (Chapter 6) and within-subjects designs (Chapter 7), those readers considering conducting a study with more than two levels of the IV or with IVs with three or more levels should refer to more specialised texts that deal with these additional issues in depth (e.g. Clark-Carter, 1997) and we would also suggest contacting a statistician for advice before proceeding.

Summary

The statistical tests in this chapter covered the analysis of the mixed-group design and introduced some new statistical concepts, these being analysis of variance (ANOVA), main effects and the interaction term. The mixed-group design represents the merger of the between-subjects and within-subjects designs and may be suitable for *some* very specific study designs. It has been seen that compared with both the between-subjects and the within-subjects *t*-tests the ANOVA for the mixed-group design is much more complicated to calculate. Fortunately, most statistical analyses for the mixed-group ANOVA and other ANOVA procedures are carried out with the aid of computer statistical packages. However, it should be borne in mind that the mixed-group design is appropriate for very specific and highly hypothesis-driven and focused studies in which an interaction term is of principal interest.

Chapter 9

Correlation and association between variables

Introduction

The experimental designs encountered thus far in this volume have, as a central tenet, the notion of manipulating one variable (IV) and measuring the effect of this manipulation on another variable (DV). This is all well and good when we have a hypothesis to test that warrants this type of experimental manipulation. However, there are some circumstances where we are not interested at all in manipulating an IV to examine the effect on a DV. Indeed, our hypothesis may merely state that there is a relationship between two variables; obviously, such a hypothesis does not automatically call for an investigative study which requires an IV manipulation. Put another way, the experimental designs that we have encountered have used an IV manipulation to determine an effect on a DV to ascertain whether there is a *causal connection* between the variables in question.

In contrast to the experimental designs outlined, *correlational* studies examine the association or relationship between two variables *but* do not imply causal connections between the variables under investigation. As such, no manipulation of an IV is required nor indeed is desirable. This is the reason that correlational studies are not in the true sense of the word experimental designs. However, correlational studies can, under the right circumstances, yield extremely valuable data *and* can be used for hypothesis testing. In the correlational study, *both* variables are measured and the association between the two variables is subjected to a statistical test of significance. The correlational study design can also provide useful findings under circumstances where it would be either impossible or unethical to conduct an experimental study, e.g. randomly allocating dialysis patients to either haemodialysis or continuous ambulatory peritoneal dialysis (CAPD) treatment modalities and examining between-groups depression for the purposes of an experimental study is likely to be rejected by every ethics committee in the UK.

Using dialysis, i.e. a treatment regime used to treat a significant proportion of renal patients in the UK, as an example, let us reconsider the notions of dialysis adequacy and depression; this was discussed earlier in Chapter 6 in relation to between-subjects designs. We know that creatinine clearance (CrCl) is implicated in renal patient survival, higher CrCl levels being generally associated with better patient outcome (Martin and Thompson, 2000b). The evidence that CrCl is related not only to mortality rates but also to more sophisticated concepts such as quality of life (Bowman and Martin, 1999) or anxiety and depression status is, however, equivocal (Martin and Thompson, 2000b). However, this is potentially a very important research question because quality of life and affective status are known to have an impact upon patient compliance to treatment. We may therefore be extremely interested to know whether there is an association between CrCl rate and self-report depression level in renal dialysis patients as this could be potentially very useful in understanding both issues of treatment compliance and adaptation to chronic illness in this patient group (Martin and Thompson, 1999). In this instance, we would measure the renal patient cohort's CrCl rate and level of depression and examine the data to determine whether higher CrCl rates were *generally* associated with lower levels of depression. This is predicting a *negative* correlation between the two variables (CrCl and depression) because we are expecting depression to be relatively *lower* with relatively *higher* levels of CrCl. It is possible to have *positive* correlations as well; for example, level of depression is known to be generally positively correlated with anxiety level, therefore *higher* levels of depression are associated with relatively *higher* levels of anxiety. It is the *strength* of the association between the two variables which we measure using the statistical test to determine whether there is a *statistically significant* relationship or association between the two variables. The criteria to determine significance level are exactly as described previously for the *experimental* designs encountered in earlier chapters, essentially a 0.05 level of significance.

A useful means of exploring the data before conducting the appropriate statistical test is to draw a *scattergram*. The scattergram represents the two variable scores for each patient where the intersection of the two scores is marked by a dot, variable one being measured on the y-axis and variable two being measured on the x-axis. Examples of scattergrams are shown in Figures 9.1–9.6.

Figure 9.1 shows a *highly* positive correlation. It can be seen that the dots are closely packed around an imaginary line representing the increase of one variable with respect to the second variable.

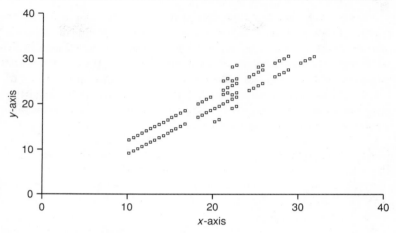

Figure 9.1 Highly positive correlation

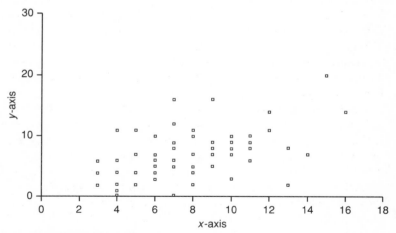

Figure 9.2 Positive correlation

Figure 9.2 shows a positive correlation; however, the correlation or association between the two variables is weaker than that in Figure 9.1. It can be seen that the dots are less closely packed around the imaginary line representing the increase of one variable with respect to the second variable.

Figure 9.3 shows a *highly* negative correlation. It can be seen that the dots are closely packed around an imaginary line representing the increase of one variable with respect to the decrease of the second variable.

Figure 9.4 shows a negative correlation; however, the correlation or association between the two variables is weaker than that shown in Figure 9.3. It can be seen that the dots are less closely packed around the imaginary line representing the increase of one variable with respect to the decrease of the second variable.

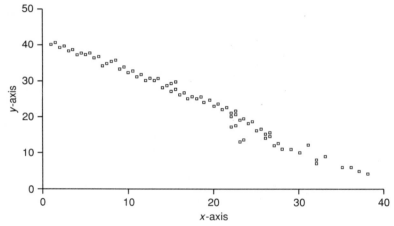

Figure 9.3 Highly negative correlation

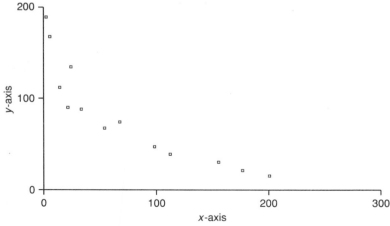

Figure 9.4 Negative correlation

Figure 9.5 shows no evidence of a correlation, there being no observed *linear* relationship between the two variables. It can be seen that the dots are randomly distributed within the frame of the scattergram.

Figure 9.6 shows the rare instance of a strong, but *non-linear*, relationship or association between two variables. In the case of a non-linear correlation being observed, the statistical tests applied to correlational data assume that the relationship between the two variables is linear, therefore it would be inappropriate to apply a statistical test to

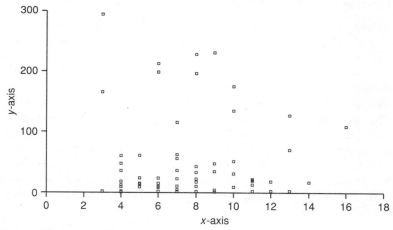

Figure 9.5 No correlation

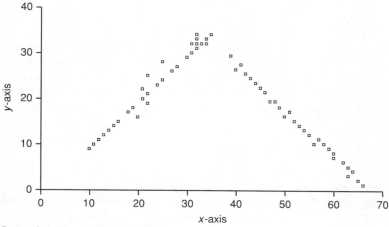

Figure 9.6 Non-linear correlation

non-linear correlational data. If a statistical test *is* applied to non-linear correlational data, a statistically significant relationship *may* be found; however, this would be erroneous to interpret and report upon. If a non-linear correlational relationship between two variables is observed, the insightful researcher should *not* conduct a statistical test but *should* report that a non-linear relationship between the two variables has been observed and present the scattergram as evidence of this.

Coefficient of correlation

The scattergram is the starting point for determining both the presence of a linear correlation (or otherwise) and the *direction* (positive or negative) of any observed correlation. A descriptive statistic known as the *coefficient of correlation* is calculated to give an index of the strength of the relationship between the two variables. This is extremely useful as it allows the strengths of a number of correlations to be compared. The coefficient of correlation statistic is represented by r. Calculation of r may be carried out by a number of statistical procedures; however, r is always measured on a scale between -1 and $+1$, where the magnitude of r represents the strength of the relationship between the two variables, i.e. the higher the value of r then the *greater* the association between the two variables. The sign indicates the direction of the association, either positive or negative.

Pearson *r*

The most common statistical test used to determine the strength of the linear correlation between two variables is the Pearson r, also known as the product–moment correlation coefficient and less frequently, although rather affectionately, as Pearson's r. Importantly, the Pearson r should *only* be used when *both* variables are of either interval or ratio level of measurement (see Chapter 2). In this respect, Pearson r should be considered as a parametric test for the analysis of correlational designs.

Calculation of Pearson *r*

Before any statistical calculation, a scattergram should be drawn to determine whether there does indeed appear to be an association between the two variables, to determine the direction of any observed relationship and, crucially, whether the association observed is linear. Having done this and confirming from the scattergram that there appears to be a linear association between the two variables, the data set should be laid out for each patient or participant. The square of each variable score for each patient is calculated, as is also a variable by variable term for each patient. The data shown relating to the renal disease hypothesis regarding a postulated relationship between CrCl and self-report depression are shown in Table 9.1 in a small cohort of ten patients.

The sum of the above tabled values for each term is then calculated thus: $\Sigma X = 960$, $\Sigma Y = 51$, $\Sigma XY = 4318$, $\Sigma X^2 = 103454$ and $\Sigma Y^2 = 333$. The calculated data are then substituted into the following formula to calculate r.

$$r = \frac{\sum XY - \dfrac{\left(\sum X\right)\left(\sum Y\right)}{N}}{\sqrt{\left(\sum X^2 - \dfrac{\left(\sum X\right)^2}{N}\right)\left(\sum Y^2 - \dfrac{\left(\sum Y\right)^2}{N}\right)}}$$

Therefore:

$$r = \frac{4318 - \dfrac{960 \times 51}{10}}{\sqrt{\left(103454 - \dfrac{921600}{10}\right)\left(333 - \dfrac{2601}{10}\right)}}$$

Table 9.1 Creatinine clearance and depression score data

Patient number	CrCl (X)	Depression (Y)	CrCl × Depression (XY)	CrCl²(X²)	Depression squared (Y²)
1	56.20	7	393.40	3158.44	49.00
2	129.30	1	129.30	16718.49	1.00
3	56.70	4	226.80	3214.89	16.00
4	150.70	3	452.10	22710.49	9.00
5	143.20	4	572.80	20506.24	16.00
6	65.90	7	461.30	4342.81	49.00
7	104.90	2	209.80	11004.01	4.00
8	84.70	8	677.60	7174.09	64.00
9	98.40	5	492.00	9682.56	25.00
10	70.30	10	703.00	4942.09	100.00

Therefore:

$$r = \frac{-578}{\sqrt{11294 \times 73}}$$
$$= -578/907.99$$
$$= -0.64$$

The critical value of r is determined by comparison of observed r with tabled r given for the 0.05 level of significance (two-tailed; Table A.7). The critical value is dependent on the number of patients/participants (N); for $N = 10$, tabled r is found to be 0.632. If observed r is equal to or greater than tabled r then it can be concluded that the relationship between the variables is statistically significant. As our observed r (-0.64) is greater than tabled r then we can conclude that there is a statistically significant negative (because a negative observed r value was obtained) correlation between creatinine clearance rate and self-report depression. Our data therefore show that self-report depression falls as creatinine clearance increases and that this relationship between the two variables is statistically significant. This finding would be reported as $r = -0.64$, $P < 0.05$. Although our hypothesis was speculatively one-tailed, the data have been analysed under the rubric of a two-tailed hypothesis because we assumed that these are data from a novel study and therefore they *could* run the very real risk of encountering a counterintuitive outcome, i.e. a significant positive correlation between the two variables. Proposing a two-tailed hypothesis under these circumstances is a good idea as we can guard against rejecting an otherwise statistically significant counterintuitive association between the two variables. The trade-off of this *statistical insurance* is that we are, in reality, specifying a slightly more conservative test statistic.

Spearman's rank order correlation (r_s)

Pearson r assumes that the two variables entered into the correlation calculation are of at least ordinal rating and also that the data satisfy a criteria of *linearity*. There are many instances in health and nursing research where at least one of the variables does not conform to an interval level of measurement. Thinking back to the pain data in Chapter 6 gives an example; this very useful and health research-appropriate DV measure was in fact at an ordinal level of measurement and would, therefore, have lacked the measurement qualities necessary to enter into a Pearson r correlational analysis. However, it is still possible to conduct a correlational analysis with data measured at the ordinal level using Spearman's rank order correlation (r_s), also referred to as Spearman's rho. Spearman's r_s tests the more general question that one variable increases as a second variable either increases or decreases. Importantly, Spearman's r_s tests this more general *monotonic* relationship or association between the two variables that does not depend on each of the variables being composed of discrete standard units. Spearman's r_s then can be considered to be a non-parametric coefficient of correlation. It is worth noting that Spearman's r_s can be used on variables that are defined by an interval or ratio level of measurement also. However, as Spearman's r_s is a non-parametric test, it less powerful than the Pearson r statistical procedure for determining significant correlational associations between two variables.

Calculation of Spearman's r_s

Before any statistical calculation involving a correlational analysis, and as we saw previously with the Pearson r analysis, a scattergram should be drawn to determine whether there does indeed appear to be an association between the two variables, to determine the direction of any observed relationship and, crucially, whether the association observed is monotonic. Having done this, and confirming from the scattergram that there appears to be a monotonic association between the two variables, the data set should be laid out for each patient or participant. The variable scores are then ranked in order from lowest to highest. In the case of tied ranks within a specific variable, each score is given the mean of the ranks that would have been allocated in the event that there had been no ties. This is a similar procedure to the non-parametric Wilcoxon analysis conducted on the within-subjects data set that was seen in Chapter 7. A differences term (D) is then calculated between each pair of ranks; D^2 is then calculated and summed. We will demonstrate this approach on the same renal data analysed by Pearson r in the previous section to illustrate that although Spearman's r_s can be used on interval or ratio data in addition to ordinal data this test is less powerful than the Pearson r procedure. Because the Pearson r data analysis was only just statistically significant at the 0.05 significance level, we may expect that the less powerful Spearman's r_s may not be able to determine a statistically significant association between the two variables. The data and accompanying calculation of D and D^2 are illustrated in Table 9.2.

The sum of D^2 (ΣD^2) therefore is 264. Spearman's r_s is then calculated by substitution of the calculated values and N (patients) in the following formula:

Table 9.2 Creatinine clearance and depression score data and ranking procedure

Patient number	CrCl	Depression	CrCl (rank)	Depression (rank)	D	D^2
1	56.20	7	1	7	−6.5	42.25
2	129.30	1	8	1	7	49
3	56.70	4	2	4	−2.5	6.25
4	150.70	3	10	3	7	49
5	143.20	4	9	4	4.5	20.25
6	65.90	7	3	7	−4.5	20.25
7	104.90	2	7	2	5	25
8	84.70	8	5	9	−4	16
9	98.40	5	6	6	0	0
10	70.30	10	4	10	−6	36

Spearman's $r_s = 1 - \{(6\Sigma D^2)/[N(N^2 - 1)]\}$

Therefore:

$r_s = 1 - \{(6 \times 264)/[10(100 - 1)]\}$

$r_s = 1 - (1584/990)$

$r_s = 1 - 1.6$

$r_s = -0.60$

The critical value of r_s is determined by comparison of observed r_s with tabled r_s given for the 0.05 level of significance (two-tailed; Table A.8). The critical value is dependent on the number of patients/participants (N); for $N = 10$, tabled r_s is found to be 0.65. If observed r_s is equal to or greater than tabled r_s then it can be concluded that the relationship between the variables is statistically significant. As our observed r_s (−0.60) is less than tabled r_s then we can conclude that there is *not* a statistically significant negative (because a negative observed r_s value was obtained) correlation between creatinine clearance rate and self-report depression. Our data therefore do not demonstrate a statistically significant association between self-report depression and creatinine clearance rate. This finding would be reported as $r_s = -0.60$, P = n.s. This example also clearly demonstrates that when compared with Pearson r, and using interval level data, Spearman's r_s is a less powerful test, and as such should be reserved specifically for data sets in which one or more of the variables is at an ordinal level of measurement.

A note on causality

Correlational studies focus on the associative dimension of variables. We have seen that experimental studies focus on manipulation of an IV (Chapters 6 and 7). However, we cannot say the same of correlational studies – we can only observe an association between two variables but cannot say whether variable one influenced variable two or whether the association was influenced by some third unencountered variable. Correlational studies therefore do not make any assumptions about causality with regard to the association between the variables under investigation *even* in the presence of a statistically significant correlation being observed.

Other uses of correlational techniques

Correlational techniques, and in particular the Pearson r statistical procedure, are extremely useful as statistical tools beyond the inferential mode of the correlational design. Pearson r is often used to determine the *test–retest reliability* of various measures. Test–retest reliability refers to how reliable an instrument is by investigating the correlations between the instrument scores after repeated administrations. This technique is used extensively in various health setting research enterprises, most notably devising and testing the properties of psychometric instruments and questionnaires.

Number of subjects required for a correlational study

In the absence of pilot data or previously published research papers, the researcher will be required to justify the minimum number of subjects required to conduct the correlational study in order to have a realistic chance of finding some statistically significant associations between variables somewhere within the data set. It has been emphasised a number of times in this volume that the researcher should make some intuitive judgement regarding the size of sample that is likely to be necessary to test the proposed hypothesis (remembering that we will not be making any predictions regarding *causality*) and detect statistically significant associations (see Chapters 4 and 5). Should the researcher be conducting a truly novel study with no available or appropriate previously published research literature to suggest minimum numbers, we would make the following recommendations as minimum subject numbers for *correlational* designs. Consistent with sample size estimations from previous chapters, the following estimations are based on power calculations (Cohen, 1988) and represent minimum subject numbers. When conducting a study in which it is predicted that there be a *medium level* of association between the two variables, the *minimum* number of subjects required for a correlational design would be eighty-five in total. When conducting a study in which it is predicted that there be a *large level* of association between the two variables, the *minimum* number of subjects required for a correlational design would be thirty in total. These estimations represent realistic *minimums* and are based on a probability $\alpha = 0.05$. We would advocate strongly that these subject numbers represent absolute *minimums* irrespective of whether the hypothesis is two-tailed or one-tailed.

Summary

This chapter introduced the correlational design and two methods of statistical analysis. The correlational design, in contrast to the experimental designs discussed in earlier chapters, explores the association or relationship between two variables in the absence of an experimental manipulation. As such, we cannot imply causality in correlational designs; all that we can say is that there is either a significant association between two variables or there is not. When both variables are of interval or ratio level of measurement, the parametric Pearson r procedure is most appropriate. Correlational studies can also be analysed using the non-parametric test Spearman's r_s if one or both variables are of an ordinal level of measurement. It has been demonstrated that the Pearson r procedure is statistically more powerful than Spearman's r_s. The utility of correlational techniques has also been discussed with regard to test retest reliability issues. The correlational design is extremely useful under circumstances where experimental manipulation of IVs may be either impossible or unethical.

Chapter 10

Single-sample studies and analysis

Introduction

The notion of a single-sample study may seem, at first, counterintuitive to the idea of quantitative and experimental research. We have seen in preceding chapters an emphasis on experimental manipulation of the IV and even in the previous chapter, which explored associations and correlations between variables without inferring causation, the importance of a comparison between two variable terms was still of paramount importance. There are, however, occasions when we may have data from a population of interest but may feel that it would be inappropriate to use a control population. These investigations are known as single-sample studies. Single-sample studies are relatively rare in the general research community, including health care research, although there is a case to advocate the design in relation to health research in which circumstances dictate that a control group is unnecessary.

Having stated this, under what circumstances would it be possible to say that a control group would be unnecessary and why may this type of design be particularly valid for health care research? The answer is that we may *already know* from the published literature what the normal or control values are for a particular DV observation. For example, the anxiety and depression data described in previous chapters were assessed using a well-known and established measure called the Hospital Anxiety and Depression Scale (HAD; Zigmond and Snaith, 1983). A normal or control set of values has been established for this measure and it has been used extensively in studies of both pathology and psychopathology (Martin and Thompson, 1999; 2000a), therefore values in relation to specific pathology have also been established. Supposing that we wanted to compare a group of cancer patients' self-report anxiety and depression levels, it may not be necessary for us to get a control group together as we could compare the cancer patients' scores against the established normal control values. On the other hand, and again using the HAD scale as an example, we may believe that we have devised a novel regime of support for our cancer patients that we would then hypothesise should result in a significant reduction of anxiety and depression in this group. We could also compare our cancer patients' scores with the published values for cancer patients who are managed and supported traditionally. In both instances, we only need to gather one sample of patients, who we could say represent a 'treatment group' or condition, and compare this group's scores statistically with control or traditionally managed and supported cancer patients' DV values on self-report anxiety and depression. This also obviously saves a great deal of time and unnecessary effort under circumstances where normative values are established. It may therefore seem that the single-sample design may be much more preferable for many purposes in health research because we will not need to be unduly concerned about a control group requirement. Although the single-sample group design is a valid approach to clinical research investigations under *some* circumstances, this type of design does, unfortunately, have some limitations.

Limitations of the single-sample design

In the true sense of the term experimentation, the single-sample study does not provide for an experimental manipulation against an IV term. Although the single-sample design compares an 'experimental group', essentially the group of patients that we have selected for study, i.e. our single sample, with a 'sham' control group, the only salient details that will be known will be the mean DV score on the variable of interest and possibly some sociodemographic data such as age or sex. What will be known about this 'group' are likely to be details on *exclusion* criteria, these being the criteria by which aberrant cases are excluded. Put simply, this means excluding all salient pathology and psychopathology except, of course, where such data are representative of the normative values for the particular pathology or psychopathology in question. Having said that, we cannot really be sure that the single sample that we have chosen is similar in patient or subject characteristics to the sample group from whom the normative values were drawn and with which the values are to be compared. Comparing this with the between-subjects design, in which patients of known category or diagnosis are randomly allocated to the two levels of the IV, we can be much more confident in this instance that the two groups are likely to be similar. There is then a higher risk of an experimental confounding effect due to some extraneous variable or characteristic of the normative value comparison group confounding our single-sample group comparison. In addition of course, should we have an idea that after the comparison we might find an unexpected result that the study may have been confounded by a patient or subject characteristic of the normative value group, we would have no redress to check the details of this group to see whether this was the case. In the worse case, we may have to design a further study, such as a between-subjects design, to ensure that we eliminate this possibility.

The exclusion criteria that are used to define the normative data are of interest because the composition and qualities of the individuals in this group uniquely define the normative value. Martin (1999) conducted a study examining locus of control (LC; Rotter, 1966) orientation in women over three phases of the menstrual cycle. The inclusion criteria that he used were exhaustive and are shown below.

Study inclusion criteria (Martin, 1999)

1   Regular menstrual cycles over the previous 6 months, an average cycle length of between 26 and 32 days, with an intercycle variability of no greater than 4 days.
2   Not taking an oral contraceptive pill for the previous 6 months or during the course of the study.
3   No current or previous history of ovarian disorders.
4   No current or previous history of depression, eating disorders or drinking problem.
5   Not currently a nursing mother.
6   Not currently dieting or dieting in the previous 6 months.
7   Not working shifts.
8   Chronic medication free.

It can be seen that the inclusion criteria are exhaustive, they also uniquely define the normative value for this group of participants, *but* how normal can we really say that this group is? To put this in perspective, the study that Martin (1999) conducted placed demands on the participants in that high levels of motivation and commitment were required. Further, as this group was all volunteers, and there would of course be many more women who fulfilled the study criteria who would not have wished to participate, we have stratified this *normal* population still further. Therefore, as an example, we may conduct a single-sample study comparing a patient population or maybe a premenstrual syndrome (PMS) population with the normative values defined by Martin (1999) for LC in normal cycling women and find a difference. However, we would have to bear in mind that normative values are derived from an extremely rigorously circumscribed group of volunteers who might be quite different and have different LC from another *normal* group of normally cycling women who perhaps did not fulfil some of the inclusion criteria or who perhaps by some undefined personality feature *do not wish* to take part in research studies.

It is an unfortunate fact of experimental design that it is extremely difficult to obtain true experimental rigour in single-sample designs because of such implicit but also occluded differences between the single-sample group and the normative value group.

A further factor that needs to be considered when deciding to use the single-sample design is that of *causation*. Single-sample designs can tell us whether there is a statistically significant difference between the sample and the normative value on some defined tacit DV measure. It is much more problematical to imply that there is a causal connection because there has been no real manipulation of an IV; at the end of the day, the researcher will be restricted to concluding *only* that there is a difference between the sample group and the normal value of another group (normative value) and there can be no summary discussion regarding what caused the observed difference.

However, having highlighted some of the more deleterious features of the single-sample design, it is useful also to provide some of this design's merits. One of the most obvious of these is the economic factor of conducting a study. The single-sample design essentially requires half the subjects of a true experimental design because we do not actually need to recruit a control or comparison group. This is obviously of great benefit where time and resource factors are of vital importance as to whether a study will actually be conducted or not. Further, we may have a *very* speculative hypothesis. This does not mean that the researcher has had a flight of fancy but rather that an original hypothesis may have come to mind, *but* because there is little published literature on the area or phenomena of interest the researcher may wish to conduct a single-sample study as a kind of pilot study to determine whether there is a difference between the sample group and normative values. The results of the single-sample study in this instance may then provide the basis for the *refinement* and *development* of an experimental hypothesis to test in a more sophisticated type of design such as an RCT. Further, the single-sample study in this scenario may be of great value in informing the researcher of the resources required to conduct the main study. This type of 'snowballing' from less sophisticated and less resource-intensive studies to more sophisticated and more resource-intensive studies is to be encouraged and also illustrates the manner in which a *research programme* may be developed.

It has to be borne in mind that, whenever the researcher chooses to use a single-sample design, what is *really* being tested is whether there is a statistically significant difference between the statistical properties and characteristics of the sample and the statistical properties and characteristics of the *normative* population. What is very clearly *not* being tested is the relationship between single sample and the normative population; in this respect, the issue of causality is not considered.

The single-sample t-test

The single-sample *t*-test is, like all *t*-tests, a parametric test and its use is subject to the parametric test assumptions outlined in Chapter 5. The single-sample *t*-test is used to compare the mean of the single sample with the normative group data mean. The rationale for the single-sample *t*-test is to examine the probability that the single-sample scores are likely to have been drawn from the same population as the normative value scores. The single-sample *t*-test assumes that at least an interval level of measurement will be used. The single-sample *t*-test is extremely useful as a test for pilot data because the statistical mechanics of the test itself do not rely on a large patient or participant population. The single-sample *t*-test can also be used when the standard deviation of the normative population sample mean is not known, making the single-sample *t*-test a very powerful but also very flexible statistical test.

A clinical example

Placing the single-sample design within an appropriate context is important, as stated earlier in the chapter. To this end, we will consider the following research question and scenario. We are interested in the locus of control (LC; Rotter, 1966) of alcohol-dependent individuals after detoxification to see whether this is different from normative values. First, however, a brief overview of LC will orientate the reader to the salient features of the LC construct and the rationale for the study design.

Locus of control primer

LC refers to a generalised expectancy of an individual's perceived control over situational factors. LC is measured on a continuum, ranging from low scores 'LC internal' to high scores 'LC external'. The general wisdom of LC research is that the more external the individual's LC then the more the same individual believes that life events are outside of his or her sphere of influence and control (Martin and Otter, 1996). Consequently, a more internal LC has been associated with better treatment outcome. The LC construct has found a psychotherapeutic niche as a measure of treatment efficacy and as a predictor of prognosis in many areas of mental health, including alcoholism (Huckstadt, 1987; Canton et al., 1988). The influence of the LC construct in relation to health research is impressive and there have been a number of derivative LC measures that have been developed over recent years, examples being the Health Locus of Control (HLC) scale (Wallston et al., 1976) and the Locus of Control of Behaviour (LCB) scale (Craig et al., 1984). An important contributing factor towards the LC being used in health settings is that it is one of the few psychological measures, easily assessed by simple questionnaire measures, that have been established to be associated with biological and disease substrates (Pfeiffer and Wetstone, 1988; Espie et al., 1990; Reynaert et al., 1995). LC orientation has also been associated with health maintenance behaviour, including breast self-examination (Nemcek, 1990).

However, because LC orientation assesses a personal belief system about control, it has been a difficult concept to relate to a behavioural outcome. This is obviously important in the case of mental health pathology and treatment evaluation. However, a dedicated LC scale designed to assess LC orientation in relation to behavioural control and a behavioural outcome has been developed and is known as the LCB scale (Craig et al., 1984). The LCB scale was devised as a means of determining control orientation before and after therapy. The LCB scale has not been used extensively, and one of the few studies that has collected normative data beyond the original validation study is that conducted by Martin (1999) and discussed briefly earlier in this chapter.

Proposed study scenario

We are interested in the LC orientation of recently detoxified alcohol-dependent individuals as we know that LC orientation is important to outcome (Canton et al., 1988). Although there are many normative LC data available, there are few relating to control of behavioural outcome. We therefore wish to use the little-used LCB measure to investigate whether our single sample of alcohol-dependent patients differs from the normative population on this measure as it relates to a behavioural outcome and could therefore be clinically useful. However, because there is little published work on the LCB measure, we take the view that perhaps it would be best to do a preliminary investigation first. This would reveal whether there is a difference in LCB orientation between the single sample and the normative population before designing and conducting a larger study with a much larger patient sample, including recruiting for a control group. We can therefore conduct a study based on a single-sample design to investigate this possibility knowing that this approach is perhaps the most resource-economic means to determine whether a further larger study is justified. Therefore, a single-sample design is used to investigate this potentially useful (but also potentially dead end) area of application of the LCB to alcohol dependency. As there are few prior data on the characteristics of the LCB measure, we will also specify a two-tailed hypothesis to take into account the possibility of significant counterintuitive findings. Although this is for the purposes of methodological rigour, it is clear to see from the data that the alcohol-dependent single sample has a greater mean LCB score than the normative sample population, i.e. the alcohol-dependent group appears to be comparatively external in LC orientation.

Computation of the single-sample t-test

The first stage in conducting the single-sample t-test is to calculate the single-sample mean LCB score of our alcohol-dependent patient cohort ($N = 18$). The mean LCB score is found to be 38.56. The standard deviation of the scores is then found to be 10.66. The calculations of the mean score and standard deviation have been described previously in Chapter 3 and will not be repeated again here.

The mean score of the normative population is then taken and is termed μ. In this example, the normative value for LCB will be taken from the follicular phase observations in Martin (1999), and therefore $\mu = 27.17$.

The single-sample mean score (X), number of patients (N), standard deviation (SD) and μ are then substituted into the following single-sample t-test formula:

$$t_{(N-1)} = \frac{\overline{X} - \mu}{SD / \sqrt{N - 1}}$$

Therefore, substituting our values we find:

$$t_{(17)} = \frac{38.55 - 27.17}{10.66/\sqrt{17}}$$

$t_{(17)} = 11.38/(10.66/4.12)$

$t_{(17)} = 11.38/2.59$

$t_{(17)} = 4.39$

The critical value of t is calculated with reference to Table A.1 with 17 degrees of freedom. As tabled t is 2.11 and calculated t is 4.39, we can conclude that there is a statistically significant difference between scores from the alcohol-dependent single sample and from the normative value. Therefore, we can conclude that the alcohol-dependent group seems to be statistically significantly more external in LC orientation, as measured by the LCB compared with the normative value. This finding would be reported as $t(17) = 4.39$, $P < 0.05$.

Conclusions from the single-sample t-test

The above example found a statistically significant difference in LCB scores between the alcohol-dependent group and the normative value. What can we conclude from this beyond the statistical inference thus described? First, we are well aware of the limitations of the design, the normative value for LCB being drawn from a study examining menstrual cycle effects on a strictly circumscribed cohort of young women. It could be more confidently concluded that we have compared a normative value for a *strictly circumscribed group* because these are all the data that we had available to conduct the comparison. Therefore, being aware of the limitations of the single-sample group design is important and should be highlighted in a study that is written up for report based on this approach. On a more positive note, what has been observed is a statistically significant difference in LCB scores, with the alcohol-dependent group being more external in LC orientation. This could be clinically a very useful finding. We have also discovered this in the most scientifically economical way possible and may therefore best use this finding as *pilot* data and indeed pilot evidence to justify a more sophisticated and ambitious main study. The logical step would in this instance be to conduct a between-subjects group comparing an alcohol-dependent male group with a *matched* non-alcohol-dependent male group. The single-sample group design is very useful for obtaining pilot data and for study and hypothesis development, it does not, however, match the rigour and robustness of the designs described in Chapters 6 and 7.

The single-sample proportions test

A limitation of the single-sample *t*-test is that it is a parametric test, although the parametric assumptions can be relaxed to analyse ordinal level data under some circumstances. There are some instances when the researcher is confronted with a nominal level of data but would still wish to carry out some analysis; this could also be under the same rubric as that of the single-sample *t*-test, such as to conduct a pilot analysis and for the purposes of further hypothesis generation and formulation. Nominal data are also extremely important and relevant in health care research. Nominal data are essential to epidemiology and can inform the researcher of issues beyond those of diagnostic category and outcome status, including giving evidence for inequity within health service resource provision.

There is, fortunately, a dedicated test for the analysis of nominal data called the single-sample proportions test. A mean score is not required for the single-sample proportions test to be performed. The single-sample proportions test procedure computes the proportion of a single sample against the proportion expected in a normal population. Therefore, only data on proportions are required for the test to be conducted. The single-sample proportions test is a non-parametric test, therefore no parametric assumptions are made regarding the data set.

A clinical example

There is a great deal of pressure on health service provision in the UK. Consider the provision of dialysis treatment for renal disease and, in particular, renal dialysis. Dialysis is an expensive treatment option, yet in patients with a diagnosis of end-stage renal disease (ESRD) some form of dialysis is essential for patient survival (Renal Association, 1997). There are two main modes of dialysis that are currently used, these being haemodialysis and continuous ambulatory peritoneal dialysis (CAPD); transplantation is a third intervention unfortunately limited by the availability of donor kidneys. Haemodialysis is more expensive than CAPD, yet there are presumed to be quality-of-life advantages for patients who are able to be dialysed using CAPD (Bowman and Martin, 1999; Martin and Thompson, 2000b). Because CAPD is still a relatively new addition to the therapeutic battery offered to ESRD patients, the characteristics of patients using this particular treatment modality may inform us a great deal about epidemiological factors in relation to renal disease. There is a great regional variation in the penetration of CAPD as a treatment modality within the UK. This may raise concerns in terms of inequities in treatment, and as regional variation has been established a conscientious researcher may wish to investigate this at a local level. Additionally, as there has been little work on sex differences in renal disease in relation to renal replacement therapy, particularly CAPD, it may therefore be a bona fide research question to investigate the possibility of sex differences in the uptake of CAPD therapy at a local level. This is for two main reasons: first, to investigate the possibility of a sex bias in accessibility to this particular treatment; second, such an investigation may inform us of other research avenues to explore if a sex difference was found. For example, we may *then* want to explore whether women come into dialysis later in the disease progression than men. The rationale for the use of the single-sample proportion test is therefore to help the researcher determine a *further* research study and *to begin to formulate* a further hypothesis. The single-sample proportions test allows the researcher to determine whether there is likely to be a research question to investigate and to do this quickly and economically. Martin and Thompson (1999) found that, in one UK centre, of the total number of ESRD patients being treated with CAPD ($N = 72$), 46 were male and 26 were female. We may expect in a normative population that half (50 per cent, or 0.5) of the patients would be expected to be women. We shall therefore take these basic data as the basis for the example computation of the single-sample proportions test.

Computation of the single-sample proportions test

The state in conducting the single-sample proportions test is to prescribe two values, these being P, the proportion of the normative population with the characteristic of interest, and p, the proportion in the single sample with this characteristic. The only other detail required to conduct the single-sample proportions test is the number of patients/participants in the single sample, which in this case would be $N = 72$. As we know that $P = 0.5$, p remains to be easily solved as follows:

p = number of female patients/N

$p = 26/72 = 0.36$

The only criterion that must be fulfilled before conducting the single-sample proportions test is that the expected numbers with or without the characteristic of interest in the single-sample group are not less than $N = 10$. The values of P, p and N are then substituted into the following formula to compute a Z score:

$$Z = \frac{p - P}{\sqrt{\dfrac{P(1 - P)}{N}}}$$

Therefore:

$$Z = \frac{0.36 - 0.5}{\sqrt{\dfrac{0.5 \times 0.5}{72}}}$$

$Z = 0.14/0.059$

$Z = 2.37$

Having calculated Z, we then refer to Table A.3 to determine the probability estimate. The probability for $Z = 2.37$ is tabled as $p = 0.0089$. As Table A.3 provides for one-tailed hypotheses and our hypothesis is essentially two-tailed, the table's probability has to be doubled and, thus, tabled $p = 0.018$. We can therefore determine that there is a statistically significant difference between our single-sample proportion compared with a normative population, $Z = 2.37$, $P < 0.05$.

Conclusions from the single-sample proportions test

The finding from the CAPD data above is interesting. The limitation of the single-sample proportions test is that there can be no *causal* connections ascribed to the data set that has been analysed. However, the finding is worthy of further investigation and can form the basis for further scientific enquiry as to why this difference exists; for example, is this related to sex-specific pathology, an inequity in health delivery or an occluded demographic characteristic? Although the single-sample proportions test makes generalisations of the findings difficult, it does, like the single-sample *t*-test, provide the foundations for both the decision to investigate this particular clinical avenue further *and* insights into the type of hypotheses to develop and the choice of methodology that we use to test these hypotheses in a proposed main study. The single-sample proportions test is particularly useful because the data that are necessary to conduct the test are usually available and accessible.

Summary

The statistical tests in this chapter cover the analysis of single-sample designs. The merits of the parametric single-sample *t*-test and the non-parametric single-sample proportions test have been described with accompanying clinical examples. Undeniably, the one-sample design is limited in terms of both the generality of findings and the lack of intrinsic methodological rigour. However, that being said, the single-sample design does have some notable benefits and merits when applied to pilot and preliminary data, and is useful for the purposes of decision making and hypothesis generation and refinement for the development of further studies which may need control groups and control treatments. In terms of time and resources, the single-sample designs are perhaps the most cost-effective designs used in quantitative research. Although currently underutilised in health research, there is much to commend the single-sample design when conducting a preliminary or pilot investigation.

Chapter 11

Confidence intervals

Introduction

Throughout this volume, the emphasis placed on the experimental designs and statistical tests to analyse them has focused very much on the notion of hypothesis testing. From this point of view, differences observed between or within groups are determined to be either statistically significant or not; there is no 'in between', the status of statistical significance being a dichotomous statement, without respect to magnitude. There has recently emerged a view that there is an overemphasis on hypothesis testing and in particular the use of P-values to determine the level of statistical significance (Gardner and Altman, 1989). These academics claim that the pursuit of understanding and interpreting study findings under the rubric of hypothesis testing and the application of a statistical test is a *limiting* factor in determining the real items of interest within the data set. Essentially, Gardner and Altman (1989) suggest that it is the *size* of the difference between groups which is important, especially in studies related to health and particularly when this is related to an outcome. Consequently, it has been suggested that these size differences are of more importance clinically than *merely* whether there is a statistically significant difference between groups as a function of the IV manipulation. Gardner and Altman (1989) have therefore advocated an alternative to such hypothesis testing to reveal more about the characteristics of the sample data, in particular how the sample data represent the larger population from which the sample was drawn. This alternative method of data description and analysis is known as *confidence intervals*.

Confidence intervals

Confidence intervals describe a range of data from the sample population and give an estimation of where the population value may lie, whether this is for a single sample, and therefore a single population, or whether, and usually more usefully, this is for two groups giving a population value for the difference based on the difference between the two compared sample scores. It is therefore important to consider confidence intervals as a measure of the precision of the sample study estimates as an index of population values. Confidence intervals have been suggested as being of great value when making inferences from the study sample with respect to the larger population from which the sample was drawn. This is obviously extremely useful in relation to health research and exploration of the usefulness of treatment effects. For example, the researcher may evaluate a novel drug treatment for cancer in a sample population and extrapolate this finding to the wider population from which the sample was drawn (i.e. all patients with the same clinical characteristics). The same logic applies for a specific nursing intervention. For example, the use of cognitive behavioural therapy (CBT) compared with cognitive analytical therapy (CAT) on treatment outcome in the mental health setting may be extrapolated from a sample group of phobic patients/clients to the whole population of phobic patients/clients from which the sample was drawn. In the general nursing setting, a comparison between a named nurse and a non-named nurse on patient satisfaction in a medical ward may be extrapolated from a sample group of medical patients to the whole population of medical patients from which the sample was drawn. A very favourable feature of the confidence interval is that within the range of values from the sample a *confidence level* can be chosen from which the researcher can conclude with this level of confidence that the population value lies. The value most often chosen for the degree of confidence is 95 per cent, although there is some debate about how useful it would be to standardise around this figure (Gardner and Altman, 1989).

The confidence interval gives an indication from a sample from a single study of the value that the researcher can expect the larger population will have within certain limits (i.e. those prescribed by the confidence interval as a function of the degree of confidence chosen, usually 95 per cent). As a general rule, the larger the width of the confidence interval then the less is the precision of the sample data in defining the population value. Two factors that can have a dramatic impact on the width of the confidence interval are, first, the size of the sample – generally, a smaller sample size corresponds to a larger width of the confidence interval and therefore less precision – and, second, the variability of the sample – the greater the variability of the sample measure then the larger the width of the confidence interval.

Extrapolating from the study sample to the population

One of the driving forces of logic in advocating the use of confidence intervals and indeed a key rationale to this approach is that sample statistics are presented as *estimates of the results that would have been obtained had the entire population been studied*. To do this, the confidence interval represents a paradigm shift from the presentation of a summary statistic, such as a group mean, and its accompanying measure of variation, such as the standard deviation, to a summary statistic that describes a range of values defined within the context of the level of confidence. Confidence intervals can be calculated for many different design types, the between-subjects and within-subjects designs being perhaps the most typical. Confidence intervals are most prevalently applied to the between-subjects design as this design type is the basis of the randomised controlled trial (RCT), the gold standard design for medical and, increasingly, nursing research.

Confidence intervals for between-subjects design

To think of the notion and calculation of confidence intervals in relation to a clinical example and the between-subjects design, we will examine the data from Chapter 6 on the between-subjects design examining the use of a new treatment for reducing the level of lipids following myocardial infarction (for an overview, see Chapter 6). The lipid level for each patient in the control and treatment groups is shown in Table 11.1. The group data required to construct the confidence interval include the mean, standard deviation and number of subjects for each group. These are shown in Table 11.2.

A 'pooled' estimate of the standard deviation is then calculated using the following formula:

$$SD = \sqrt{\frac{(N_1 - 1)S_1^2 + (N_2 - 1)S_2^2}{N_1 + N_2 - 2}}$$

Therefore:

$$SD = \sqrt{\frac{(10 - 1)1.35^2 + (10 - 1)1.73^2}{18}}$$

Table 11.1 Lipid level as a function of group type

Group 1 (control/placebo) ($N_1=10$) (X_1)	Group 2 (treatment) ($N_2=10$) (X_2)
5	3
3	4
5	2
5	2
7	6
6	7
8	4
6	6
5	3
6	4

Table 11.2 Data required to calculate a confidence interval

Index	Control group	Treatment group
Mean	5.6	4.1
Standard deviation	1.35	1.73
Number of patients	10	10

Therefore:

$$SD = \sqrt{\frac{16.38 + 26.94}{18}}$$

Therefore, pooled SD = 1.55.

The standard error (SE) of the difference between the two group means is then calculated thus:

$$SE_{diff} = SD \times \sqrt{\frac{1}{N_1} + \frac{1}{N_2}}$$

Therefore:

$$SE_{diff} = 1.55 \times \sqrt{\frac{1}{10} + \frac{1}{10}}$$

$$SE_{diff} = 0.69.$$

Generally, to construct the confidence interval at a level of confidence of 95 per cent, it is necessary to utilise the central 95 per cent of the normal distribution. Therefore, the extreme values of the normal distribution (5 per cent) are required to be removed, these values representing the two extremes of each tail of the distribution and representing 2.5 per cent of the normal distribution in each tail. It is worth remembering that confidence interval analysis is invariably used in the *two-tailed* sense, therefore both tails of the normal distribution are removed to conduct the analysis. Specifically, because the calculation of confidence intervals in relation to the between-subjects design examines the difference between sample means, the *t*-distribution is used as the sampling distribution. A $100(1 - \alpha)$ per cent confidence interval is initially constructed and this equates to the following calculation of the confidence interval itself:

difference between sample means $- (t_{1 - \alpha/2} \times SE_{diff})$ to

difference between sample means $+ (t_{1 - \alpha/2} \times SE_{diff})$

$t_{1 - \alpha/2}$ is taken from the *t*-distribution with $N_1 + N_2 - 2$ degrees of freedom (Table A.1). In this case, a 95 per cent degree of confidence with 18 degrees of freedom = 2.101. Therefore, the confidence interval is calculated thus:

$1.5 - (2.101 \times 0.69)$ to $1.5 + (2.101 \times 0.69)$

Therefore, the 95 per cent confidence interval for these data is calculated to be 0.05 to 2.95. Importantly, this calculation of the confidence interval is describing the values that we would expect the *population* scores to fall into with 95 per cent confidence.

Confidence intervals for within-subjects design

Confidence intervals can be readily calculated for within-subjects designs where there are two levels of the IV. Indeed, the calculation of the within-subjects design confidence interval is even more simple than the calculation used for the between-subjects calculation described above. To think of the notion and calculation of confidence intervals in relation to a clinical example and the within-subjects design, we will examine the data from Chapter 7 on the within-subjects design, examining the change in patient anxiety scores after admission to hospital following MI between time of admission and day 5 of admission (for a review of this study, see Chapter 7). In addition to the mean difference score, to calculate a within-subjects confidence interval, a difference standard

Table 11.3 Anxiety score at admission and day 5 post MI and difference score calculation

Patient number	On admission (X_1)	Day 5 of admission (X_2)	d $(X_1 - X_2)$
1	5	3	2
2	3	3	0
3	5	4	1
4	5	2	3
5	4	3	1
6	11	2	9
7	11	8	3
8	11	3	8
9	6	2	4
10	9	4	5

deviation score is required to be calculated. The data and difference score are shown in Table 11.3.

The mean difference between scores on day 1 and on day 5 is calculated to be 3.6. The standard deviation of the difference scores is found to be 2.99. The SE is then calculated as follows:

$$SE = SD \text{ of differences}/\sqrt{N}$$

Therefore:

$$SE = 2.99/\sqrt{10}$$

$$SE = 0.95$$

In this case, a 95 per cent degree of confidence with $(N-1)9$ degrees of freedom = 2.262. Therefore, the confidence interval is calculated thus:

$$3.6 - (2.262 \times 0.95) \text{ to } 3.6 + (2.262 \times 0.95)$$

Therefore, the 95 per cent confidence interval for these data is calculated to be 1.45 to 5.75. Importantly, this calculation of the confidence interval is describing the values that we would expect the *population* scores to fall into with 95 per cent confidence.

Reporting confidence intervals in scientific reports

Confidence intervals are easily incorporated into the results section of clinical research studies. The result of the study described above would be reported as $t(9) = 3.82$, $P < 0.05$; mean difference in anxiety 3.9, 95 per cent confidence interval 1.45 to 5.75. There is a preference among some journals to emphasise the confidence interval before the statistical test result, however this approach is not universally accepted and it is still appropriate and acceptable to quote the statistical test before the confidence interval.

Utility of confidence intervals

Confidence intervals can be calculated for a large variety of design types used in health research that have been included in this volume, e.g. confidence intervals can be calculated for correlational and regression designs and for comparisons between sample proportions and odds ratios. The method of calculation is similar across most design types and specialised texts are available (e.g. Gardner and Altman, 1989) which cover the mathematics in question in far greater detail than space allows here.

The use of confidence intervals

Confidence intervals are easily calculated and allow the researcher to make an inference about the characteristics of the patient group participating in the study with respect to the larger population from which the study sample was drawn. There are now a number of journals which report health research which expect confidence intervals to be used in describing the study findings, the *British Medical Journal* (BMJ) is among these. However, a number of those researchers who advocate the use of confidence intervals down play the value of hypothesis testing and the use of statistical tests; we believe this practice should be discouraged. There are certainly a large number of journals that will be orientated towards hypothesis testing in the conduct and reporting of findings, this inevitably requires a formal statistical analysis to be carried out. A rational view is to use confidence intervals *in addition* to the reporting of statistical differences and within the context of hypothesis testing. Taken together, the use of hypothesis testing and confidence intervals adds to the value and interpretation of a study because both are powerful tools for exploring the data.

Summary

Confidence intervals add another exciting tool to the health researcher's armamentarium of techniques and provide the opportunity to gain further insights into the data collected from a research study. Confidence intervals allow the researcher to make inferences with a level of confidence from the study sample with respect to the clinical population from which the study sample was drawn. Contrary to the opinion of a few health researchers, confidence intervals are not a replacement for hypothesis testing and the application of statistical tests. Confidence intervals can be used to inform the reader of a published study with more detail, but this should only be, in our view, in addition to the reported hypothesis and reported statistical test of significance.

Chapter 12

Graphical presentation of data

Introduction

Having conducted a study, the findings will need to be presented for a report of some kind. Indeed, there are a number of routes through which the data and findings may be presented, such as a local report, a peer-reviewed journal article or a conference presentation. Whatever the context of the report, the clarity and accessibility of the findings are of paramount importance. An important technique for displaying study data in an accessible way is through the use of effective data presentation, using the most appropriate graphical technique. A further useful way of summarising data, which will be considered later in this chapter, is by means of a summary table.

Data graphics

Presenting data graphically does more than simply replace a summary table of means and standard deviations. There is no doubt that key *statistical* material should always be presented in some form of summary table, this is particularly true when some kind of statistical analysis has been conducted on the data. Further, a summary table of means and associated standard deviations is of great use to those reading the research report because these data can be used to calculate the power of the study and the patient/participant numbers required for a replication study to be conducted. Therefore, graphical data presentation is *not* a substitute for a summary table, which is essential. The strength of presenting data graphically is that the medium itself is intrinsically accessible and easily understood to the reader. In this sense, presenting data graphically *adds* to the report in terms of an additional quality of clarity. This is the case of course only if the data presented graphically are presented *well*. It is worth remembering that the whole idea of presenting data graphically is to add to the understanding and accessibility of the research report. Therefore, whenever a graphical description of findings is used in a report, the graphical presentation *must* be firmly referred to and anchored within the text.

Fundamentals of data presentation

A fundamental tenet in informing the choice of graphical presentation technique is to base this on the study design and analysis, with particular attention to the level of measurement. As a general rule, data measured at the nominal or ordinal level are presented with graphics that explicitly state the data values, the rationale for this being that these levels of measurement are of discrete (nominal) or ordered (ordinal) categories. This gives a wide choice of data presentation types and includes tables, bar charts and pie charts. Data measured at the interval or ratio level are of a continuous nature, and the presentation techniques used generally reflect this quality of continuity. The most suitable presentation media for these types of data are histograms (essentially, a bar chart with defined and continuous axes), line graphs, these being particularly useful for the presentation of within-subjects design findings, and scattergrams, the preferred technique for describing graphically data from correlational design studies.

User-friendly graphical presentations

Tufte (1983) reviewed the characteristics of graphics which enhanced and detracted from a presentation. The negative aspects described by Tufte (1983) are more or less the opposite of each of the positive points made. Therefore, for the purposes of brevity, the following represent the main points in Tufte (1983) in ensuring graphical presentations are as user friendly, non-confusing and accessible as possible:

- use full words (not abbreviations), do not use complex codes;
- brief explanations for clarification;
- labels placed on the graphic;
- clear typeface;
- lines are thin and contrasts are used only to emphasise changes in data measures;
- graphics should be 50 per cent wider than they are tall.

We would also add to this by suggesting that the researcher avoids the use of three-dimensional graphics as these detract from a presentation, incur a loss of transparency in the data and are generally not well received by peer-reviewed journals and their reviewers.

Keeping within the boundaries of the above guidelines will produce clear and useful charts which will enhance the overall presentation of the research findings. An example of a good graphical presentation of data in the form of a pie chart is shown in Figure 12.1.

An example of a good graphical presentation of data in the form of a bar chart is shown in Figure 12.2. Examples of good graphical presentation of data in the form of a correlational chart have been illustrated in Chapter 9.

Summary tables

The presentation of key data in a summary table is a key element in ensuring a research study is accessible. Background details on the characteristics of the patient/participant population are usefully summarised in such a table. Summary tables are often used to summarise the DV mean scores and associated standard deviations as a function of the IV manipulation. In this way, a summary table can also provide the reader with a clearer insight into the experimental design used. A further crucial feature of a summary table of DV means and standard deviations is that a reader can use these summary figures to calculate the statistical

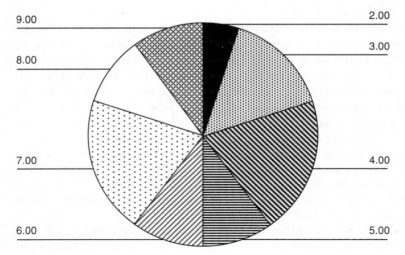

Figure 12.1 Pie chart

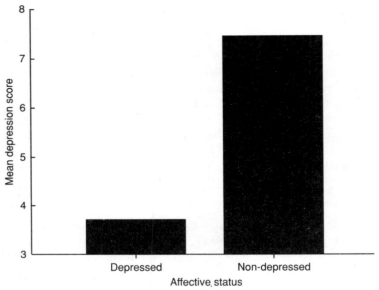

Figure 12.2 Bar chart

power of the study and, in the event that no statistically significant effect of IV manipulation was observed, the sample size that is likely to be required to observe a statistically significant difference as a function of the IV manipulation in planning a future replication study.

Summary tables should always be presented simply and clearly, usually with the relevant mean scores and associated standard deviations (SD). The description of the table should also be as clear and concise as possible. Table 12.1 shows a good example of a summary table taken from the study on end-stage renal disease by Martin and Thompson (1999) that was used to describe important characteristics of the patient population under investigation.

This summary table displays a great deal of information about the clinical group in an unambiguous manner. Because all of the measures are circumscribed by a unique unit, a column has been added to describe the unit details. Where the unit of each variable is uniform and has been described clearly in the methodology section of the report, it is not necessary to restate this in the summary table. An example of this is shown in the following summary table (Table 12.2) from the same study (Martin and Thompson, 1999) which describes the levels of anxiety and depression within the same unit context.

Table 12.1 Demographic and clinical data

Variable	Unit	Mean	SD
Age	(years)	51.36	14.63
Time on CAPD	(months)	23.47	23.26
Kt/V	(weekly)	2.03	0.41
Body surface area	(m²)	1.81	0.20
Serum albumin	(g/l)	35.04	3.81
Serum haemoglobin	(g/dl)	10.66	1.41
Water generation	(l/24 h)	1.72	0.77
Estimated total body water	(l)	37.56	6.52
Weight	(kg)	71.84	14.79
Height	(cm)	168.08	9.05
Serum urea	(mmol/l)	20.49	5.54
Creatinine clearance	(l/week/1.73 m²)	71.97	25.04
Serum creatinine	(μmol/l)	896.42	286.85
Residual renal function	(ml/24 h)	710.78	818.68

Table 12.2 Mean scores and standard deviations (SD) of patients' scores on psychometric measures

Variable	Mean	SD
HAD Total	12.14	6.26
HAD-A Anxiety subscale	6.90	3.76
HAD-D Depression subscale	5.24	3.51

It was stated earlier that a summary table of the means and SDs can also inform the reader of salient details of the study's experimental design, particularly where these are clearly circumscribed by the IV within the same summary table. This approach also allows a summary of the statistical analysis to be included as well as associated significance levels. The summary table below (Table 12.3) from a recent study on the effect of manipulating diet on mood state (Martin and Bonner, 2000) serves as an illustration of these points. The variable measures listed are all described in their full and abbreviated forms in the original paper and, within this context, it is appropriate to use the abbreviated term within the summary table. All the measures are self-report indices of anxiety or depression using the same units.

Close examination of the summary table reveals there to be three levels of the IV, which in this case is diet type (control/carbohydrate/protein); the methods section of the paper states that the investigation used a within-subjects design; the layout of the data in the summary table allows the reader to visualise and understand the study design with ease. Exact *P*-values are quoted because the statistical analysis in this instance was

Table 12.3 Affective state measures as a function of dietary manipulation, associated *F*- and *P*-values (standard deviations are shown in parentheses)

Variable	Control	Carbohydrate	Protein	F-value	P-value
HAD-A	12.06 (4.65)	11.11 (4.81)	11.50 (4.93)	0.73	0.49
HAD-D	6.94 (3.08)	6.28 (3.51)	7.17 (3.13)	1.12	0.34
STAI-T	52.67 (14.36)	51.00 (13.78)	52.39 (13.86)	0.77	0.47
STAI-S	46.22 (11.73)	46.88 (14.61)	47.83 (13.24)	0.46	0.64
BDI	18.83 (7.60)	15.44 (8.21)	17.06 (7.97)	2.60	0.09
LCB	38.56 (10.66)	37.65 (12.16)	39.56 (10.53)	0.33	0.72

carried out by a computer program (SPSS) that gives exact *P*-values (Chapter 13).

Summary

This chapter briefly described the principles of good data presentation using a graphical medium. Certain types of chart lend themselves more readily to the presentation of different types of data, the level of measurement being one of more important aspects to consider when deciding which type of graphical presentation to use. Summary tables are also of great importance in describing the important features of data, particularly the means and the standard deviations. Summary tables are useful for describing the clinical characteristics of the patient population under investigation. Summary tables are also useful for reporting the results of a statistical analysis, particularly where a number of DVs are being measured and compared as a function of the IV manipulation.

Chapter 13

The use of computers for statistical analysis

Introduction

The experimental designs and statistical analyses described in this volume are easy to conceptualise and, with practice and familiarity with the statistical formulas, the statistical component can be readily calculated. An interesting and useful innovation over recent years has been the development of computer-based statistical programs.

Evolution of computer-based statistical analysis

Originally, computer-based statistical programs were targeted at specialist mathematicians and statisticians and an understanding of machine code computer program languages such as PASCAL, COBOL and C was extremely desirable as required knowledge if the user was to use the programs properly and effectively. Needless to say, at that point, few researchers were using computer-based statistical programs in the health care setting and their use, such as it was, was focused on audits and epidemiology. In summary, these early computer-based statistical programs were user unfriendly and accessible only to specialists. Therefore, the potential usefulness of these programs to health research had yet to be realised.

Attempts were then made to development computer-based statistical programs that were more user friendly and did not require specialist programming knowledge to be able to run the statistical analysis successfully. The rationale of this was that these programs would have a wider market and could be introduced into niche areas and disciplines, such as psychology and biostatistics, which had a strong statistical component but which did not have mathematicians or statisticians. An example of this was the introduction of the statistical programs for the social sciences (SPSS). One of the early versions of SPSS was known as SPSS-X and this was designed to operate on a large mainframe computer accessible by a terminal; although this represented a vast improvement over earlier programs, the fact that the program required a large mainframe computer for operation restricted its use somewhat, particularly to those institutions which had a mainframe computer. The next innovation was the development of SPSS-PC+, which as the acronym suggests was developed to be run on the personal computer (PC). Obviously, developing the program for use on the PC was an enormous improvement in terms of accessibility and allowed much wider utilisation of the program. Although this SPSS-PC+ became widely used as an accessible and useful computer-based statistical program, there still remained an issue or difficulty. This difficulty was a limitation of the user interface; essentially, the way in which the user interfaced with the computer program. SPSS-PC+ operated with the computer-operating system Microsoft DOS (MSDOS). This limitation made SPSS-PC+ somewhat difficult and unwieldy to use for the *occasional* user of the program, such as a psychologist or nurse researcher. The next logical step that was taken to deal with this aspect of usability was to develop the program for the Microsoft Windows operating system. When SPSS for Windows was introduced, a watershed in computer-based statistical programs was reached. SPSS for Windows was easy to use because it extensively utilised the Microsoft Windows environment by means of a graphical user interface (GUI). Data became extremely easy to enter, code, transform and manipulate with this development, and the statistical tests were simply chosen from a menu and then executed with a click of the mouse. SPSS for Windows has thus become the leading computer-based statistical program which can be used to conduct a large variety of statistical tests, including all those covered in this book. The success of SPSS for Windows can be evaluated by a number of factors, not least by the number of revisions and upgrades for the program that have been developed over recent years to further increase its power. In addition, an examination of peer-reviewed journals reporting quantitative analysis will reveal that many of the studies have used SPSS for Windows in the conduct of the data analysis. There are many other computer-based statistical programs that have followed a similar developmental pathway to SPSS for Windows and that also offer the health researcher much in terms of statistical power and ease of operating: BMDP and MINITAB, to name just two. However, SPSS for Windows is the most popular and widely used program and provides a useful example in describing the evolutionary causeway of computer-based statistical analysis developments.

The use of computer-based statistical programs to the health researcher

There is little doubt that the advent of computer-based statistical programs has been a great boon to the health researcher. The ease of use of such programs coupled with the ability of these programs to analyse more sophisticated experimental designs has allowed health researchers to explore hitherto inaccessible research design questions and, consequently, to develop more sophisticated research hypotheses. The fact that these analyses can be conducted at the touch of a mouse button, having chosen the test from a test menu, is also an important time advantage compared with conducting the statistical tests by hand, even with the aid of a calculator. The example of the mixed-group study (Chapter 8) and the rather lengthy process by hand of conducting the statistical analysis will give some indication of how useful the time-saving aspect of the computer-based statistical package can be to the health researcher. Consequently, we are great advocates of the use of the computer-based statistical analysis package and believe that the use of such programs should be more widely endorsed. A recent paper on renal disease illustrates this point. The paper on the quality of life of patients with end-stage renal disease treated with continuous ambulatory peritoneal dialysis (CAPD) (Martin and Thompson, 2000b) demonstrates a fairly sophisticated statistical analysis using a technique called *multiple regression*. Martin and Thompson (2000b) conducted a large number of these analyses because this type of statistical analysis was central to addressing the research question. These analyses were conducted using SPSS FOR WINDOWS and took a few moments to calculate. Had these statistical analyses been conducted by hand, it is fair to say that this would have taken the best part of a *whole day* to complete. One final advantage of computer-based statistical programs is that they give an exact value for significance, e.g. $P = 0.023$. In this sense, computer-based statistical programs can be perceived as being more accurate than statistical calculations conducted by hand.

Limitations of computer-based statistical programs to the health researcher

A number of very good reasons to apply computer-based statistical programs to the analysis of data sets have already been pointed out. There are, however, some limitations to these programs, some of which are based on the program itself and others on the skills and knowledge base of the *user of the program*. The limitations of the program itself are based on the fact that, given the data and an instruction to conduct a test, the program will perform some kind of analysis and produce some kind of result. It will not, however, tell the researcher if they have selected the *right* test to be conducted. A wrong test may have been selected, yet the programs will still be likely to carry out the test and produce an erroneous but plausible set of results. This could obviously be a disaster to the researcher wishing to write up findings for a journal paper or a conference presentation.

This is less likely to happen if the researcher conducts the analysis using pencil and paper because the data are laid out for calculation in such a way that it is easy to determine the design type and also easy to spot whether there is an error or anomaly in the data and then recalculate. Because the computer-based statistical program *does not* give a step-by-step account of how the data are being manipulated, it is very difficult to determine whether there is an error in the data or, indeed, in the data manipulation. There are *some* computer-based statistical programs which will give an indication, under some circumstances, that the wrong test has been selected; BMDP does this, but most statistical programs will only report an error if the program itself cannot make sense of the data (which is rare).

The skills and knowledge base of the user are also a factor that can limit the usefulness of the computer-based statistical program. First, there is the example described above; basically, the selection of the wrong test. A second factor is the *data input* into the statistical program worksheet; this has to be carried out both *meticulously* and *correctly*. Data can be entered in the wrong format or with errors. In both instances, even in the event of the correct test being conducted, the result will be *wrong*. A further, more insidious, factor is that reliance on the computer-based statistical package can make the researcher rusty, very quickly, on the complexities of experimental design. It has been seen throughout this volume that the choice of statistical test is a function of the design type and vice versa. Therefore, if the researcher conducts an analysis by hand, this give an added insight into the characteristics of the design that they have chosen, the rationale for the choice and also a *sensitivity to the data*. This dimension is certainly missing if the researcher never conducts tests by hand, and this can lead to both errors in data analysis and errors in the *interpretation* of the findings. Additionally, it is also possible to carry out very sophisticated statistical analyses using the computer programs described. This is of great importance and contribution when used *appropriately*. However, it is important to consider whether there is a rationale for using a very sophisticated data analysis.

It has been stressed throughout this volume that the main thrust of designing a research study is to address a *research question*. The research question *must* be based on a defined research hypothesis. It cannot be stressed enough that the best research hypotheses are the most *simple* ones, although they are unlikely to explain complex phenomena. Extrapolating this to the research design then, the best design type will be the most simple because it will be based on a simple readily designed hypothesis. This is part of the reason why RCTs are known as the 'gold standard' for research designs, particularly in relation to clinical trials.

There are many instances that the authors are aware of where researchers have conducted extremely complicated analyses *because the computer will do it* rather than because the experimental design called for it. These studies are generally *poor* in quality and *ambiguous* in the presentation and interpretation of the findings. The power of the computer-based statistical program can therefore encourage the naïve researcher to conduct a sophisticated and inappropriate statistical analysis and this practice should be avoided. A useful way to think about this particular issue is to think principally about the experimental hypothesis and the design type at all times. It is also worth thinking about how the test could be conducted by hand; if the researcher knows that the test cannot be computed by hand, then it is good policy to consider whether the planned analysis by the computer-based statistical program is, *in reality*, the most appropriate and contextually sensitive to the research hypothesis. The best advice in deciding on an experimental design and the type of data analysis, whether this is to be conducted by hand or by computer, is *keep it simple*.

Summary

This chapter introduced the development and use of computer-based statistical programs for conducting analysis. It has been highlighted that computer-based statistical programs are a useful aid to the researcher and the use of such programs is advocated and endorsed. Computer-based statistical programs have also been seen to be very useful in terms of the researcher's time constraints as tests can be conducted very quickly indeed compared with calculations by hand, even with the aid of a calculator. There are some limitations in the use of computer-based statistical programs and these largely focus on the fact that most of the programs will conduct an analysis even if the wrong type of test is selected. Second, the use of such programs can encourage researchers to use more sophisticated types of statistical analysis than is usually required.

On balance, computer-based statistical packages have much to offer the health researcher, but in order for these computer packages to be used most effectively the researcher must remain in touch with the fundamentals of experimental design.

Chapter 14

Considerations when designing a clinical study

Introduction

The experimental designs and statistical analyses described thus far will cover the majority of issues of clinical enquiry which can be investigated using a quantitative methodology. However, it is important to be aware that a constellation of other factors are encountered when designing a study to investigate health issues and when using patients in a general nursing setting or clients in a mental health setting as participants in a study. A number of these issues are concerned with the well-being of the participant, such as consent, confidentiality and anonymity. A further important issue, and one that is not often discussed within study design and analysis texts, is the medical–legal aspects of conducting a study. These include issues of researcher accountability and researcher and institutional indemnity or insurance. Studies can go wrong, and this is especially true of clinical trials using newly developed drugs whose pharmacological properties are being explored in humans for the first time. There are other unforeseen circumstances that may have an impact upon a study half-way through to completion. Examples of these will be given later, but can range from overestimating the willingness of the patient group to participate to wrangles with other members of the multidisciplinary team, usually, but not exclusively, doctors.

Ethics

It may seem that stating that a study should be ethical is an obvious prerequisite to the conduct of clinical studies and, of course, this is true. However, the term ethics can seem rather nebulous, so it seems worthwhile to explore a little deeper the notion of conducting an ethically acceptable study. Nurses enjoy a very special relationship with patients, a relationship based on trust, care and unconditional positive regard. The patient sees the nurse as a *nurse* not as a researcher, therefore when conducting a study the nurse will have to ensure that these qualities of the nurse–patient relationship are not compromised by the procedures involved in conducting the study. Given this, it is also important to ensure that these very positive aspects of the nurse–patient relationship do not bias the investigations and result in erroneous findings. An example of this is the concept of *social desirability* and social desirability bias.

Social desirability

A nurse may be conducting a study on patients' perception of pain. If the nurse conducting the study is known to the patient, it may well be possible that the patient will give a biased answer when the nurse assesses the level of pain. This is because the patient knows the nurse, they have a good relationship and the patient may feel that they want to be regarded and evaluated by the nurse positively. In this sense, the patient may report less pain than they are in fact feeling because they may feel that reporting a high level of pain (which they are indeed experiencing) would be a disappointment to the nurse. A way around this is to identify a nurse to conduct the study who is not known to the patients under investigation. Under these conditions, the patients are less likely to respond with a social desirability bias.

The notion of minimal risk

A further key issue in conducting ethically acceptable research is the notion of *minimal risk*. The keystone to conducting ethical research is to achieve the highest ratio of benefit to risk, and a crucial part of this is careful planning and design of the study. Risk must be minimised as much as possible, and the term minimal risk is used to denote that the study should not incur an elevated risk to the experimental or treatment group compared with the control group. Part of minimising any risk is to make sure that the literature that supports the conduct of the study and the experimental hypotheses is thoroughly reviewed. This prevents the most unfortunate of circumstances where a study has begun to be conducted and *then* it is discovered that another similar study has been published and that the study the researcher is conducting is little more than a replication. Replication studies are of course appropriate under some circumstances, indeed the scientific method that is applied to conducting the type of studies outlined in this volume is based on the notion that the methodology is rigorous enough for a replication to be conducted. However, if the researcher has planned to do a *novel* investigation, it is no excuse to find out half-way through the study that the study is not novel at all; this type of replication is entirely unnecessary and places an unfair additional burden on the patients who have consented to take part.

Conduct

Interactions involving patients should always be conducted courteously and with due respect, and nurses engaging in a research study should, in this regard, commit to these ideals of interaction throughout the research process. Additionally, the research nurse may need to give reassurance and support to patients beyond the immediate defining parameters of the study and should be prepared to accept and carry out this duty. Patients may be anxious about their performance or may have questions unrelated to the immediate conduct of the study. In these circumstances, the research nurse should give appropriate support and guidance. It should always be remembered that the nurse who is engaged in a research project *remains* professionally accountable and responsible for their conduct and practice. One grim reality of conducting research that is sometimes encountered is that of *boredom*. If the nurse conducting the research is administering the same test, questionnaire or procedure over and over again to patients, it is entirely possible that the nurse could become bored. This is acceptable and to be expected under some circumstances. What is not acceptable is to communicate this boredom to the patient; therefore, in this instance, and where feasible, take a break and come back to the procedural session refreshed and cheerful!

Ethical committees and the Declaration of Helsinki

The care of patients participating in research studies is of paramount concern and is, in fact, part of international law, with ethical guidelines determined by the Declaration of Helsinki. Although the Declaration of Helsinki is couched very much in terms of medical research conducted by physicians, the basic tenets of the declaration are applied to health research in a clinical setting. The main thrust of the Declaration of Helsinki is to preserve the rights, choices and care of patients. This includes the notion of minimum risk but also the notion of informed patient consent, discussed later.

Whenever a study is designed that is going to be using patients in research, an application has to be made to the local ethics committee, which will give a recommendation as to whether the study is indeed ethically sound. The local ethics committee, which comprises health professionals and, usually, at least one lay representative, often a local member of the community health council, may ask for revisions to the study before ethical approval is given. Depending on the composition of the committee members, the committee may give some advice on study design aspects too. It is not entirely unusual for the ethics committee to ask the researcher to a meeting to discuss the study proposal further.

Informed consent

A critical part of the study is that of obtaining informed consent from the patient. Typically, this means explaining the study to the patient in detail and highlighting what the expectation of the patient would be in participating in the study. The experimental hypotheses should not be disclosed to the patient, however, as this may influence a bias in the findings and invalidate any results. The patients will usually give written consent and sign a consent form to say that the study has been explained to them, that they are aware of any risks involved and that they are willing to participate. Patients are always advised that they can withdraw from a study at any time and this is usually written into the text of the consent form.

Confidentiality and anonymity

Patients should always be assured that their participation in the study is confidential. This means that the researcher will not reveal to others what has been observed in *individual* patients. If patients are to be followed up, then it is usual to code the data and data collection tools in such a manner that a patient's identity is not revealed to anyone who may come across a data form. The usual way of achieving this is to use code numbers with an identifier sheet kept *separately* in a secure place. If patients are not followed up then of course they can remain anonymous.

Trust approval and trust indemnity

Having gained ethical approval to conduct the study, the researcher should approach the research and development office of the NHS Trust (presuming the study is being conducted within this context) for formal permission from the Trust to conduct the study. The researcher should ensure that when such permission is given this also includes Trust indemnity. Trust indemnity is an insurance which will ensure that the Trust, ather than the individual researcher, is held accountable for the investigation r should anything go wrong during the course of the study and a patient wishes to complain or even sue.

Professional rivalries

Professional rivalry can become an issue that can have an impact on the conduct of a nurse-led research study and can have a lasting effect on the relationships among members of the multidisciplinary team. Interestingly, we had not planned to include the issue of professional rivalry in this volume until we encountered it first hand during a recent investigation. We will give our experience as an example and let the reader draw their own conclusions and, indeed, moral of the tale. We were conducting a study on quality of life in renal disease patients undergoing CAPD (see Chapter 6). A relatively small amount of funding had become available to support the study and to employ a research nurse part-time for a year.

Having designed the study, we approached the renal consultants by letter with an overview and asked for an opinion because we planned to use patients who were under their care as participants. A number of small concerns were raised and one of us (C.M.) attended a ward meeting to talk the study through with the ward team, including the consultants, and the study was agreed by all concerned after a questionnaire was dropped from the study protocol. It is fair to say that, although the consultants showed some interest in the study, it was fairly clear to all concerned that they did not really want to be involved in the study themselves but were happy to give permission to approach their patients as participants. The study was conducted and two feedback sessions were held to give a preliminary overview of the findings to the ward team, including the consultants. These sessions received good feedback and participation from all concerned. About 6 months after completion of the study, C.M. received a letter from one of the consultants asking 'how the analysis of the study was going?' C.M. replied that the analysis had gone very well and that a research paper had been written up *and* accepted for publication in a leading *psychology* journal. Next, a reply letter arrived from the same consultant *complaining* that they (the consultants) had not seen the manuscript and given *their* comment and approval before submission and asking what acknowledgement *they* had in the paper in terms of authorship. C.M. despatched a reply to the consultant saying that the consultant had received an acknowledgement in the paper *for support* but had not been included as an author as the consultant did not fulfil the criteria for authorship (see below); the consultants had not contributed to the paper or to the study at all in terms of being partners in research, they had merely given permission to approach their patients for consent. It is fair to say that the other two consultants did not have a problem with this and one in particular was very pleased that papers were coming out from the study. Why did this situation arise? We can only speculate, although part of the reason may be the journal that accepted the publication; perhaps the consultant in question may not have kicked up a fuss had the paper been accepted in the *Nursing Times* as opposed to a leading psychology or medical journal. The other factor is an interesting feature of medical doctors and publications. Some consultants would appear to believe that the status of consultant is the only criterion for being cited as an author on a research report, this is not of course the case. Indeed, this practice is clearly unacceptable and unethical and should be discouraged. It certainly does not in any conceivable way fulfil the criteria for authorship. The reader is invited to draw his or her own conclusions from our experience.

Authorship rights and publication

The above example of professional rivalry issues gives an indication of the importance of knowing basic rights and guidelines in relation to the authorship of scientific papers from a study for publication. The main criterion for being an author on a paper, and that generally agreed by most academic institutions, is that an individual *must* have made a significant contribution to *writing* the paper to qualify as an author; this does not of course include proof-reading or commenting on a completed draft. A further criterion often set in addition to contributing to writing the paper is that the researcher must have made a significant contribution to designing and conducting the study. Collecting data on behalf of the person who designed the study would not qualify as authorship. Some guidelines also suggest that to qualify for authorship, particularly in multiauthor studies, the researcher must have a reasonable understanding of all aspects of the study including those which may not be of their special interest, e.g. all authors should understand why a particular statistical analysis was chosen even though only one of the authors may have conducted the analysis.

The researcher who contributed most to the conduct of the study is usually the first-mentioned author. Academic supervisors are usually named last in the authorship list. Where all authors have made a more or less equal contribution to the paper, authorship is usually arranged in alphabetical order (on surnames). Those who do not satisfy the criteria for authorship but have helped with the study in some way are usually mentioned by name in an acknowledgements section at the end of the paper – see Martin and Bonner (2000), Martin and Thompson (1999) and Martin and Thompson (2000b) for examples. There are also rare but important circumstances under which it is appropriate to dedicate a paper, usually but not exclusively following the death of a colleague or research collaborator; for examples, see Martin (1999) and Thompson and de Bono (1999).

Time constraints

There is no doubt that the conduct of a study will invariably be time consuming. Researchers are often overoptimistic about their investigation timetables and there are a number of reasons for this. It should be mentioned that any proposed investigation should have a timetable of milestones to cover the research enterprise. This is an extremely important aspect of good research practice. The timetable will indicate to the researcher whether the research schedule is on course and whether any remedial action is necessary. Quite often, researchers will devise a timetable that covers just the conduct of the study itself. This is generally bad practice because it does not build in time for writing up the findings, which can be very time consuming, particularly if a further review of some of the literature is required or if additional source literature has to be ordered. Often, unforeseen events occur during a study which delay its progress. These can range from low numbers of patients recruited onto the study to the researcher becoming ill; the list of possibilities is endless. In view of this, we would suggest that, in addition to the estimated time to conduct and complete the study, an additional stretch factor in terms of time of a *minimum* of 50 per cent should be added.

Funding

A study will need some kind of resource initiative in order to be conducted. Even the smallest studies which may be conducted in nurses' spare time will incur some kind of cost. However, even when conducting a relatively modest study, some form of additional support and resource provision might be required. This if often achieved by a research grant which will cover part or all of the associated costs of the planned investigation, often including the researchers' overheads. Competition for research grants is quite fierce, although there are many grant-funding bodies prepared to support nursing research initiatives. These include the Department of Health, the Research Councils, charities and pharmaceutical and health care companies. When an application to a grant-awarding body is made, the awarding body will usually wish to see a full study proposal and associated costings. Following the submission of the application, the awarding body will meet and make a decision on funding. This process can take several months and can be a source of stress to the applicant who has a study 'ready to go' but who is waiting on an unknown committee to decide whether the investigation will be supported. We would suggest that the researcher should be calm but should also design more than one study and apply for funding from other research-funding bodies. This gives the best possible chance of securing the required support for a planned investigation.

Summary

This chapter has given a broad overview of ancillary issues which are important to address and be aware of when designing and conducting an investigation. These factors range from ethical issues and the importance of informed consent, interdisciplinary relationships and authorship to logistical and funding issues. The importance of ensuring that the researcher has formal Trust indemnity before conducting the study cannot be overstated. Dissemination of research findings is critically important both to developing evidence and to improving clinical practice in nursing; the issue of ensuring appropriate recognition in terms of paper authorship is therefore of great importance academically. Having an awareness of these factors and their invaluable role in and contribution to the completion of a successful study will go a long way to ensuring that the research investigation is both an interesting and *enjoyable* process.

Appendix: Statistical tables

Table A.1 The t-distribution

Critical values of t (two-tailed). In the case of a one-tailed test, the significance levels must be divided by 2.

	Significance level	
d.f.	0.10	0.05
1	6.314	12.706
2	2.920	4.303
3	2.353	3.182
4	2.132	2.776
5	2.015	2.571
6	1.943	2.447
7	1.895	2.365
8	1.860	2.306
9	1.833	2.262
10	1.812	2.228
11	1.796	2.201
12	1.782	2.179
13	1.771	2.160
14	1.761	2.145
15	1.753	2.131
16	1.746	2.120
17	1.740	2.110
18	1.734	2.101
19	1.729	2.093
20	2.086	2.086
21	1.721	2.080
22	1.717	2.074
23	1.714	2.069
24	1.711	2.064
25	1.708	2.060

Table A.1 continued

26	1.706	2.056
27	1.703	2.052
28	1.701	2.048
29	1.699	2.045
30	1.697	2.042
40	1.684	2.021
60	1.671	2.000
120	1.658	1.980
∞	1.645	1.960

Notes
Abridged from © 1963 R. A. Fisher and F. Yates. Reprinted with permission from Addison Wesley Longman Limited, reprinted with permission from Pearson Education Limited.

Table A.2 The Mann–Whitney test

The critical values are presented for U (two-tailed) at a significance level of 0.05. In the instance of a one-tailed test, the presented values are significant at the 0.025 level.

N_2 \ N_1	5	6	7	8	9	10	11	12	13	14	15	16	17	18	19	20
5	2	3	5	6	7	8	9	11	12	13	14	15	17	18	19	20
6		5	6	8	10	11	13	14	16	17	19	21	22	24	25	27
7			8	10	12	14	16	18	20	22	24	26	28	30	32	34
8				13	15	17	19	22	24	26	29	31	34	36	38	41
9					17	20	23	26	28	31	34	37	39	42	45	48
10						23	26	29	33	36	39	42	45	48	52	55
11							30	33	37	40	44	47	51	55	58	62
12								37	41	45	49	53	57	61	65	69
13									45	50	54	59	63	67	72	76
14										55	59	64	67	74	78	83
15											64	70	75	80	85	90
16												75	81	86	92	98
17													87	93	99	105
18														99	106	112
19															113	119
20																127

Table A.3 Z-test table

Critical values for one-tailed test. In the instance of a two-tailed test, the probability estimates should be doubled.

Z	0.00	0.01	0.02	0.03	0.04	0.05	0.06	0.07	0.08	0.09
0.0	0.5000	0.4562	0.4222	0.4483	0.4443	0.4404	0.4364	0.4325	0.4286	0.4247
0.2	0.4207	0.4168	0.4129	0.4090	0.4052	0.4013	0.3974	0.3936	0.3897	0.3859
0.3	0.3821	0.3783	0.3745	0.3707	0.3669	0.3632	0.3594	0.3557	0.3520	0.3483
0.4	0.3446	0.3409	0.3372	0.3336	0.3300	0.3264	0.3228	0.3192	0.3156	0.3221
0.5	0.3085	0.3050	0.3015	0.2981	0.2946	0.2912	0.2877	0.2843	0.2810	0.2776
0.6	0.2743	0.2709	0.2676	0.2643	0.2611	0.2578	0.2546	0.2514	0.2483	0.2451
0.7	0.2420	0.2389	0.2358	0.2327	0.2296	0.2266	0.2236	0.2206	0.2177	0.2148
0.8	0.2119	0.2090	0.2061	0.2033	0.2005	0.1977	0.1949	0.1922	0.1894	0.1867
0.9	0.1814	0.1841	0.1788	0.1762	0.1736	0.1711	0.1685	0.1660	0.1635	0.1611
1.0	0.1587	0.1562	0.1539	0.1515	0.1492	0.1469	0.1446	0.1423	0.1401	0.1379
1.1	0.1357	0.1335	0.1314	0.1292	0.1271	0.1251	0.1230	0.1210	0.1190	0.1170
1.2	0.1151	0.1131	0.1112	0.1093	0.1075	0.1056	0.1038	0.1020	0.1003	0.0985
1.3	0.0968	0.951	0.0934	918	0.0901	0.0885	0.0869	0.0853	0.0838	0.0823
1.4	0.0808	0.0793	0.0778	0.0764	0.0749	0.0735	0.0721	0.0708	0.0694	0.0681
1.5	0.0668	0.0655	0.0643	0.0630	0.0618	0.0606	0.0594	0.0582	0.0571	0.0559
1.6	0.0548	0.0537	0.0526	0.0516	0.0505	0.0495	0.0485	0.0475	0.0465	0.0455
1.7	0.0446	0.0436	0.0427	0.0427	0.0418	0.0409	0.0401	0.0392	0.0375	0.0367
1.8	0.0359	0.0351	0.0344	0.0336	0.0329	0.0322	0.0314	0.0307	0.0301	0.0294
1.9	0.0287	0.0281	0.0274	0.0268	0.0262	0.0256	0.0250	0.0244	0.0239	0.0233

x	.00	.01	.02	.03	.04	.05	.06	.07	.08	.09
2.0	0.0228	0.0222	0.0217	0.0212	0.0207	0.0202	0.0197	0.0192	0.0188	0.0183
2.1	0.0179	0.0174	0.0170	0.0166	0.0162	0.0158	0.0154	0.0150	0.0146	0.0143
2.2	0.0139	0.0136	0.0132	0.0129	0.0125	0.0122	0.0119	0.0116	0.0113	0.0110
2.3	0.0107	0.0104	0.0102	0.0099	0.0096	0.0094	0.0091	0.0089	0.0087	0.0084
2.4	0.0082	0.0080	0.0078	0.0075	0.0073	0.0071	0.0069	0.0068	0.0066	0.0064
2.5	0.0062	0.0060	0.0059	0.0057	0.0055	0.0054	0.0052	0.0051	0.0049	0.0048
2.6	0.0047	0.0045	0.0044	0.0043	0.0041	0.0040	0.0039	0.0038	0.0037	0.0036
2.7	0.0035	0.0034	0.0033	0.0032	0.0031	0.0030	0.0029	0.0028	0.0027	0.0026
2.8	0.0026	0.0025	0.0024	0.0023	0.0023	0.0022	0.0021	0.0021	0.0020	0.0019
2.9	0.0019	0.0018	0.0018	0.0017	0.0016	0.0016	0.0015	0.0015	0.0014	0.0014
3.0	0.0013	0.0013	0.0013	0.0012	0.0012	0.0011	0.0011	0.0010	0.0010	0.0010
3.1	0.0010	0.0009	0.0009	0.0009	0.0008	0.0008	0.0008	0.0008	0.0007	0.0007
3.2	0.0007									
3.3	0.0005									
3.4	0.0003									
3.5	0.00023									
3.6	0.00016									
3.7	0.00011									
3.8	0.00007									
3.9	0.00005									
4.0	0.00003									

Table A.4 Chi-square (χ^2) test

Critical values for chi-square test (two-tailed) at 0.05 level of significance.

d.f.	0.05 level of significance
1	3.84
2	5.99
3	7.82
4	9.49
5	11.07
6	12.59
7	14.07
8	15.51
9	16.92
10	18.31
11	19.68
12	21.03
13	22.36
14	23.68
15	25.00
16	26.30
17	27.59
18	28.87
19	30.14
20	31.41
21	32.67
22	33.92
23	35.17
24	36.42
25	37.65
26	38.88
27	40.11
28	41.34
29	42.56
30	43.77

Notes
Abridged from © 1963 R.A. Fisher and F. Yates. Reprinted
with permission from Addison Wesley Longman Limited.
Reprinted with permission from Pearson Education Limited.

Table A.5 Wilcoxon test

The critical values for T (two-tailed) at 0.05 level of significance. In the instance of a one-tailed test, the significance levels must be divided by 2.

N	0.05 level
6	0
7	2
8	4
9	6
10	8
11	11
12	14
13	17
14	21
15	25
16	30
17	35
18	40
19	46
20	52
21	59
22	66
23	73
24	81
25	89

Table A.6 F-values for analysis of variance (ANOVA) at 0.05 level of significance (one-tailed)

Degrees of freedom in denominator	Degrees of freedom in numerator														
	1	2	3	4	5	6	7	8	9	10	15	20	30	60	120
1	161.40	199.50	215.70	224.60	230.30	234.00	236.80	238.90	240.50	241.90	245.90	248.00	250.10	252.20	253.30
2	18.51	19.00	19.16	19.25	19.30	19.33	19.35	19.35	19.38	19.43	19.43	19.45	19.46	19.48	19.49
3	10.13	9.55	9.28	9.12	9.01	8.94	8.89	8.85	8.81	8.79	8.70	8.66	8.62	8.57	8.55
4	7.71	6.94	6.59	6.39	6.26	6.16	6.09	6.04	6.00	5.96	5.86	5.80	5.75	5.69	5.66
5	6.61	5.79	5.41	5.19	5.05	4.95	4.88	4.82	4.77	4.74	4.62	4.56	4.50	4.43	4.40
6	5.99	5.14	4.76	4.53	4.39	4.28	4.21	4.15	4.10	4.06	3.94	3.87	3.81	3.74	3.70
7	5.59	4.74	4.35	4.12	3.97	3.87	3.79	3.73	3.68	3.64	3.51	3.44	3.38	3.30	3.27
8	5.32	4.46	4.07	3.84	3.69	3.58	3.50	3.44	3.39	3.35	3.22	3.15	3.08	3.01	2.97
9	5.12	4.26	3.86	3.63	3.48	3.37	3.29	3.23	3.18	3.14	3.01	2.94	2.86	2.79	2.75
10	4.96	4.10	3.71	3.48	3.33	3.22	3.14	3.07	3.02	2.98	2.85	2.77	2.70	2.62	2.58
11	4.84	3.98	3.59	3.36	3.20	3.09	3.01	2.95	2.90	2.85	2.72	2.65	2.57	2.49	2.45
12	4.75	3.89	3.59	3.36	3.11	3.00	2.91	2.85	2.80	2.75	2.62	2.54	2.47	2.38	2.34
13	4.67	3.81	3.41	3.18	3.03	2.92	2.83	2.77	2.71	2.67	2.53	2.46	2.38	2.30	2.25
14	4.60	3.74	3.34	3.11	2.96	2.85	2.76	2.70	2.65	2.60	2.46	2.39	2.31	2.22	2.18

15	4.54	3.68	3.29	3.06	2.90	2.79	2.71	2.64	2.59	2.54	2.40	2.33	2.25	2.16	2.11
16	4.49	3.63	3.24	3.01	2.85	2.74	2.66	2.59	2.54	2.49	2.35	2.28	2.19	2.11	2.06
17	4.45	3.59	3.20	2.96	2.81	2.70	2.61	2.55	2.49	2.45	2.31	2.23	2.15	2.06	2.01
18	4.41	3.55	3.16	2.93	2.77	2.66	2.58	2.51	2.46	2.41	2.27	2.19	2.11	2.02	1.97
19	4.38	3.52	3.13	2.90	2.74	2.63	2.54	2.48	2.42	2.38	2.23	2.16	2.07	1.98	1.93
20	4.35	3.49	3.10	2.87	2.71	2.60	2.51	2.45	2.39	2.35	2.20	2.12	2.04	1.95	1.90
25	4.24	3.39	3.10	2.87	2.71	2.60	2.51	2.45	2.39	2.35	2.20	2.12	2.04	1.95	1.90
30	4.17	3.32	2.92	2.69	2.53	2.42	2.33	2.27	2.21	2.16	2.10	1.93	1.84	1.74	1.68
40	4.08	3.23	2.84	2.61	2.45	2.34	2.25	2.18	2.12	2.08	1.92	1.84	1.74	1.64	1.58
60	4.00	3.15	2.76	2.53	2.37	2.25	2.17	2.10	2.04	1.99	1.84	1.75	1.65	1.53	1.47
120	3.92	3.07	2.68	2.45	2.29	2.17	2.09	2.02	1.95	1.91	1.75	1.66	1.55	1.43	1.35

Table A.7 Product–moment correlation coefficient for parametric correlations

The critical values for the product–moment correlation coefficient in calculation of Pearson's r at 0.05 level of significance.

N	0.05 level of significance
3	0.997
4	0.950
5	0.878
6	0.811
7	0.754
8	0.707
9	0.666
10	0.632
11	0.602
12	0.576
13	0.553
14	0.532
15	0.514
16	0.497
17	0.482
18	0.468
19	0.456
20	0.444
21	0.433
22	0.423
23	0.413
24	0.404
25	0.396
26	0.388
27	0.381
28	0.374
29	0.367
30	0.361

Table A.8 Spearman's r_s non-parametric correlation test

The critical values of r_s at a significance level of 0.05. In the instance of a one-tailed test, the significance levels should be divided by 2.

N	0.05 level of significance
5	1.00
6	0.89
7	0.79
8	0.74
9	0.68
10	0.65
11	0.61
12	0.59
13	0.56
14	0.54
15	0.52
16	0.51
17	0.49
18	0.48
19	0.46
20	0.45
21	0.44
22	0.43
23	0.42
24	0.41
25	0.40
26	0.39
27	0.38
28	0.38
29	0.37
30	0.36

Notes
Abridged from © 1963 R. A. Fisher and F. Yates. Reprinted with permission from Addison Wesley Longman Limited. Reprinted with permission from Pearson Education Limited.

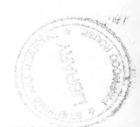

References

Beck, A. T., Ward, C. H., Mendelson, M., Mock, J. and Erbaugh, J. (1961) 'An inventory for measuring depression', *Archives of General Psychiatry* 4, 561–571.

Bowman, G. S. and Martin, C. R. (1999) 'Evidence of life quality in CAPD patients and implications for nursing care: a systematic review', *Clinical Effectiveness in Nursing* 3, 112–123.

Canton, G., Giannini, L., Magni, G., Bertinaria, A., Cibin, M. and Gallimberti, L. (1988) 'Locus of control, life events and treatment outcome in alcohol dependent patients', *Acta Psychiatrica Scandinavica* 78, 18–23.

Clark-Carter, D. (1997) *Doing Quantitative Psychological Research: From Design to Report* (Psychology Press, Hove).

Cohen, J. (1988) *Statistical Power Analysis for the Behavioral Sciences* (Lawrence Erlbaum Associates, Hillsdale, NJ).

—— (1992) 'A power primer', *Psychological Bulletin* 112, 155–159.

Craig, A. R., Franklin, J. A. and Andrews, G. (1984) 'A scale to measure the locus of control of behaviour', *British Journal of Medical Psychology* 57, 173–180.

Department of Health (1991) *Research for Health. A Research and Development Strategy for the NHS* (Department of Health, London).

—— (1999) *Making a Difference. Strengthening the Nursing, Midwifery and Health Visiting Contribution to Health and Healthcare* (Department of Health, London).

Espie, C. A., Gillies, J. B. and Montgomery, J. M. (1990) 'Anti-epileptic polypharmacy, psychosocial behaviour and locus of control orientation among mentally handicapped adults living in the community', *Journal of Mental Deficiency Research* 34, 351–360.

Gardner, M. J. and Altman, D. G. (1989) *Statistics with Confidence* (British Medical Journal, London).

Huckstadt, A. (1987) 'Locus of control among alcoholics, recovering alcoholics, and non-alcoholics', *Research in Nursing and Health* 10, 23–28.

Martin, C. R. (1999) 'Phasic influences on psychometric measures during the menstrual cycle: implications for the construct integrity of the locus of control dimension', *British Journal of Medical Psychology* 72, 217–226.

Martin, C. R. and Bonner, A. B. (2000) 'A pilot investigation of the effect of tryptophan manipulation on affective state in male chronic alcoholics', *Alcohol and Alcoholism* 35, 49–51.

Martin, C. and Otter, C. R. (1996) 'Locus of control and addictive behaviour', in A. B. Bonner and J. Waterhouse (eds) *Addictive Behaviour: Molecules to Mankind*, pp. 121–134 (Macmillan, London).

Martin, C. R. and Thompson, D. R. (1999) 'Utility of the Hospital Anxiety and Depression Scale in patients with end-stage renal disease on continuous ambulatory peritoneal dialysis', *Psychology, Health and Medicine* 4, 369–376.

—— (2000a) 'A psychometric evaluation of the Hospital Anxiety and Depression Scale in coronary care patients following acute myocardial infarction', *Psychology, Health and Medicine* 5, 193–201.

—— (2000b) 'Prediction of quality of life in patients with end-stage renal disease', *British Journal of Health Psychology* 5, 41–55.

Martin, C. R., Bowman, G. S., Knight, S. and Thompson, D. R. (1998) 'Progress with a strategy for developing research in practice', *Nursing Times Research* 3, 28–34.

Martin C. R., Bowman, G. S. and Thompson, D. R. (2000) 'The effect of a coordinator on cardiac rehabilitation in a district general hospital', *Coronary Health Care* 4, 17–21.

Meddis, R. (1984) *Statistics Using Ranks* (Blackwell Scientific Publications, Oxford).

Nemcek, M. A. (1990) 'Health beliefs and breast self-examination among black women', *Health Values, Health Behavior, Education and Promotion* 14, 41–52.

Otter, C. R. and Martin, C. R. (1996) 'Personality and addictive behaviour', in A. B. Bonner and J. Waterhouse (eds) *Addictive Behaviour: Molecules to Mankind*, pp. 87–120 (Macmillan, London).

Pfeiffer, C. A. and Wetstone, S. L. (1988) 'Health locus of control and well-being in systemic lupus erythematosus', *Arthritis Care and Research* 1, 131–138..

Renal Association (1997) *Treatment of Adult Patients with Renal Failure: Recommended Standards and Audit Measures,* 2nd edn (Royal College of Physicians, London).

Reynaert, C., Janne, P., Bosly, A., Staquet, P., Zdanowicz, N., Vause, M., Chatelain, B. and Lejeune, D. (1995) 'From health locus of control to immune control: internal locus of control has a buffering effect on natural killer cell activity decrease in major depression', *Acta Psychiatrica Scandinavica* 92, 294–300

Rotter, J. B. (1966) 'Generalised expectancies for internal versus external control of reinforcement', *Psychological Monographs* 80.

Siegel, S. (1956). *Nonparametric Statistics for the Behavioral Sciences* (McGraw-Hill, New York).

Thompson, D. R. (1998) 'The art and science of research in clinical nursing', in B. Roe and C. Webb (eds) *Research and Development in Clinical Nursing Practice* (Whurr, London).

—— (1999) 'Making nursing research visible' (Guest editorial) *Nursing Times Research* 4, 325–326.

Thompson, D. R. and de Bono, D. P. (1999) 'How valuable is cardiac rehabilitation and who should get it?', *Heart* 82, 545–546.

Tufte, E. R. (1983) *The Visual Display of Quantitative Data* (Graphics Press, Cheshire, CT).

Uuskula, M. (1996) 'Psychological differences between young male and female survivors of myocardial infarction', *Psychotherapy and Psychosomatics* 65, 327–330.

Wallston, B. S., Wallston, K. A., Kaplan, G. D. and Maides, S. A. (1976) 'Development and validation of the health locus of control (HLC) scale', *Journal of Consulting and Clinical Psychology* 44, 580–585.

Zigmond, A. and Snaith, R. P. (1983) 'The Hospital Anxiety and Depression Scale', *Acta Psychiatrica Scandinavica* 67, 361–370.

Index